Transformative Nursing
in the NICU

Mary E. Coughlin, RN, MS, NNP, founder and president of Caring Essentials Collaborative, LLC, has served as their global learning officer since 2010. Ms. Coughlin's seminal work merging The Joint Commission concept of core measures with developmentally supportive care frames her current passion. Author of the 2011 National Association of Neonatal Nurses "Guidelines for Age-Appropriate Care of the Premature and Critically Ill Hospitalized Infant" in addition to other publications, Ms. Coughlin is an internationally recognized expert in the field of trauma-informed age-appropriate care and cultural transformation in the NICU.

Ms. Coughlin's clinical background spans over 30 years, with a focus on neonatal nursing and advanced practice as a neonatal nurse practitioner at the Brigham & Women's Hospital, Boston, Massachusetts. A graduate of Northeastern University, where she received her baccalaureate and Master of Science degrees, Ms. Coughlin also served as an officer in the United States Air Force Nurse Corps for 7 years. Those who have heard her speak describe Ms. Coughlin as motivational and transformational.

Transformative Nursing
in the NICU

Trauma-Informed Age-Appropriate Care

MARY E. COUGHLIN, RN, MS, NNP

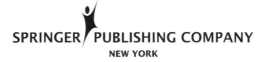

SPRINGER PUBLISHING COMPANY

NEW YORK

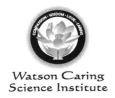

Watson Caring
Science Institute

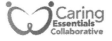

Springer Publishing Company, LLC
11 West 42nd Street
New York, NY 10036
www.springerpub.com

Acquisitions Editor: Elizabeth Nieginski
Composition: Newgen Imaging

ISBN: 978-0-8261-9657-6
e-book ISBN: 978-0-8261-9658-3

14 15 16 / 5 4 3 2 1

The author and the publisher of this Work have made every effort to use sources believed to be reliable to provide information that is accurate and compatible with the standards generally accepted at the time of publication. Because medical science is continually advancing, our knowledge base continues to expand. Therefore, as new information becomes available, changes in procedures become necessary. We recommend that the reader always consult current research and specific institutional policies before performing any clinical procedure. The author and publisher shall not be liable for any special, consequential, or exemplary damages resulting, in whole or in part, from the readers' use of, or reliance on, the information contained in this book. The publisher has no responsibility for the persistence or accuracy of URLs for external or third-party Internet websites referred to in this publication and does not guarantee that any content on such websites is, or will remain, accurate or appropriate.

Library of Congress Cataloging-in-Publication Data
Coughlin, Mary, author.
  Transformative nursing in the NICU: trauma-informed age-appropriate care / Mary Coughlin.
      p. ; cm.
  Includes bibliographical references and index.
  ISBN 978-0-8261-9657-6—ISBN 978-0-8261-9658-3 (e-book)
  I. Title.
  [DNLM: 1. Neonatal Nursing—methods. 2. Family Health. 3. Infant, Newborn—psychology. 4. Intensive Care, Neonatal—psychology. 5. Neonatal Nursing—standards. 6. Stress, Psychological—nursing. WY 157.3]
  RJ253.5
  618.92'01—dc23

                                                                                                          2013038837

Printed in the United States of America by Gasch Printing.

This book is dedicated to all the premature and critically ill infants and their families across the globe. May the information in this book provide clinicians and administrators with the necessary research and evidence to transform the experience of care in the neonatal intensive care unit, and, in doing so, transform the outcomes of this incredibly fragile patient population.

To quote Dr. Seuss: "Sometimes the questions are complicated and the answers are simple." The answer is care, to care consistently and reliably with every patient encounter.

Contents

Foreword

*T*his work about the neonatal intensive care unit (NICU) offers a doorway to all areas of health care delivery in that it highlights and explores in depth the global issues of quality, vulnerability, medical harm, and risks of hospitalization—even with the best of intentions, system goals, and mission.

Human factors often contribute to trauma and affect age-appropriate care, which author Mary E. Coughlin develops with a depth of scholarship within the context of whole-system considerations. She also addresses the history and evolution of a consciousness of adverse events and negligence that occurs in hospitalized patients and families. This consciousness of adverse events and negligence affects not only patients, families, and communities, but also care providers.

This history and reality of adverse effects and the inherent risks of hospitalization are explored against the backdrop of nursing's legacy of human caring in the NICU. To help address these service-delivery constraints and mishaps, Ms. Coughlin offers core measures for how to overcome, if not transform, the variables affecting quality, age-appropriate caring.

By highlighting the dynamics and priorities of basics that have been nursing's domain across time, core measures are introduced: for example, the nurse's role in the healing environment; protecting sleep; age-appropriate activities of daily living; prevention and management of pain and stress; and family-centered caring. These measures are antidotes to human and system errors; nursing can provide distinctive leadership to implement these changes. However, nursing and systems alike require an advanced knowledge base, informed by ethics and evidence of best practices including multiple forms of knowledge, which offer another way forward for nursing care in the NICU.

The core remedies offered in this work are guided by concrete nursing exemplars; they are universal and global in perspective. These remedies hold the promise of shifting a culture of error into an authentic, informed culture of care to ensure safety and "carefulness."

Finally, Mary E. Coughlin implores nurses with a call to action to create and transform current practices. These include the future of health care in the NICU for prevention and whole person/family care, affecting human as well as social systems.

Jean Watson, PhD, RN, AHN-BC, FAAN
Distinguished Professor and Dean Emerita
University of Colorado Denver, College of Nursing
Founder, Watson Caring Science Institute
www.watsoncaringscience.org

Preface

I am truly honored and grateful for the opportunity to have written this book. In looking back over the past year, I never imagined that the concept of trauma-informed age-appropriate care in the neonatal intensive care unit (NICU) would resonate so profoundly with neonatal clinicians across the globe.

Although I have been a passionate crusader and evangelist of developmentally supportive care for some time, linking this approach to care with the experience of developmental trauma has been transformational. I was introduced to the concept of trauma-informed care during a brief but profound clinical experience as the interim nurse manager of an inpatient adolescent psychiatric unit. Having had no psychiatric nursing experience (outside of nursing school), I was, to say the least, apprehensive about taking on this role. I was blessed to receive the support and mentorship of several amazing psychiatric nursing experts who facilitated my role transition and expanded my understanding of inpatient psychiatric nursing.

As part of my orientation, I attended a 2-day training session titled "A Nonlinear Dynamics Approach to Sensory Modulation," presented by Tina Champagne, OTD, OTR/L, CCAP, with several of my psych colleagues. The content was a revelation in understanding the concept of trauma and how sensory experiences could modulate and even provide a level of healing for the trauma survivor.

My aha moment—this was the NICU!

Galvanized with this new knowledge, I began to look at the NICU experience through a trauma lens. I voraciously read everything I could get my hands on related to trauma, developmental trauma, neurobiology of stress, and the vulnerability and susceptibility of the premature and critically ill infant to medical trauma.

It became vividly obvious that neonatal clinicians and hospital administrators *must* dramatically change the existing paradigm associated with neonatal intensive care. So I began blogging on the subject (http://quantumcaring.blogspot.com) and presenting at various national and international conferences, introducing the concept of trauma-informed age-appropriate care, as well as providing evidence-based care strategies aimed at mitigating and minimizing the toxic stress associated with intensive care hospitalization.

When Elizabeth Nieginski from Springer Publishing Company contacted me, I was excited to share with her the work I had been doing; I was not expecting her to invite me to write a book. My writing experiences were limited to blogging and a few journal articles of which I was a coauthor. A book, *wow*, that was a big deal and I knew I would need support. I am honored by this opportunity and grateful for all the support, patience, and guidance Elizabeth has given me over this past year.

Funny how you don't know what you don't know, and writing a book, well…it has been an amazing, humbling, insightful learning journey. As I look back on the experience and review the content, I hope the information presented inspires and informs, but, more importantly, translates into clinical practice.

The Quality Caring Institute of Caring Essentials Collaborative, LLC, is an online learning site supported by Moodle, an open-source virtual learning environment. For more information about Moodle, please visit their site: https://moodle.org/about.

To access the companion learning resources to this book, you must create a login before proceeding to the online learning resources. To begin, go to http://moodle.caringessentials.org and select login and then register. Guest login will not give you access to the learning materials. Once you have registered, select the course titled "Transformative Nursing in the NICU" and enroll using the enrollment key TNN2014. Please share your feedback and constructive comments regarding this web-based learning experience at contact@caringessentials.org.

Mary E. Coughlin

Acknowledgments

There is nothing new under the sun, and the opportunity to write this book and reframe the concepts of developmentally supportive care is only possible through the work of many dedicated professionals who have preceded me. That being said, I would like to formally express my gratitude to Nan Stromberg, Tina McCarthy, and Beverly Moore, who supported and mentored me as the interim nurse manager of the adolescent psychiatric unit at Carney Hospital, Dorchester, Massachusetts. Your clinical expertise and compassion were profoundly inspiring; I couldn't have done the job without you and certainly would not have written this book without that experience.

Sharyn Gibbins and Steve Hoath, my coauthors on the original paper, titled "Core Measures for Developmentally Supportive Care"—your collaboration, expertise, and insights in framing the core measures created the template for the work in this book. Thank you.

National Association of Neonatal Nurses (NANN), thank you for the opportunity in 2011 to translate the core measures into the national guidelines for age-appropriate care of the premature and critically ill hospitalized infant—with a special thank you to Diane Galazzo for recommending me to the NANN board to work on this project.

Alison Grant, Ana Garcia, Anna Kalber, Chrissie Israel, Esmeralda Molina, Francoise Guyomard, Sara Russell, Therese Vasconcellos, and Thomas Kuehn, I want to thank you guys especially for your passion, your friendship, your constructive criticism, and your validation of the precepts underpinning this book. In corroborating the challenges of neonatal clinicians to provide trauma-informed age-appropriate care regardless of geographic location, your insights authenticate the universality of the evidence-based care strategies presented in this book. Thank you, *obrigada, danke, gracias,* and *merci.*

To Danny—what can I say? First the dictation software: I know I was a bit resistant at first, but am super-appreciative of your admonishments and encouragement to use this resource and streamline my workflow. Most importantly, I would not be sitting here today writing this Acknowledgment without your belief in me to succeed, to jump and dive into my passion, to leave a good-paying steady job and follow my heart. Ever since that moment I have never looked back and have never been happier. Thank you doesn't seem sufficient; you are the BEST.

Last but not least, I want to express my deepest gratitude to my family. To my children Tara, Sean, Britt, Sammi, Alex, and Hayley: the constancy of your support, your motivational text messages, Facebook likes, and love—143.

SECTION I: *Quality Health Care: Global Initiative*

CHAPTER 1: *Quality Health Care*

Quality in a service is not what the provider puts in.
It's what the customer gets out.—Peter F. Drucker

In 2001, the Institute of Medicine's (IOM) landmark publication *Crossing the Quality Chasm: A New Health System for the 21st Century* exposed the U.S. health care system's glaring quality and safety deficits. On the heels of its 1999 publication, *To Err Is Human: Building a Safer Health System,* which exposed the gross fallibility of the system and the need to reduce preventable medical error, the IOM made an urgent call to action for system redesign directed to health care professionals, health care policymakers, consumer advocates, regulatory agencies, and general health care consumers.

Quality in health care is a global initiative. Dramatic advances in medical technology, pharmaceuticals, genomics, and surgical interventions have enabled health care professionals to save more lives than ever before. With these cutting-edge strategies comes enormous responsibility at the individual and system levels to ensure patient safety and quality in service.

FIRST DO NO HARM

The concept of "first do no harm" has its origins in ancient medicine, dating back to the Egyptian physicians in 2400 BCE and reaffirmed during the time of Hippocrates—400 BCE. This credo of nonmaleficence continues into modern health care as an ethical and moral priority. "First do no harm" for nurses emanates from Florence Nightingale's early work and her famous publication, *Notes on Nursing,* articulating the role and duties of the nurse. "It may seem a strange principle to enunciate as the very first requirement in a hospital that it should do the sick no harm" (Nightingale, 1863, Preface). Despite the primacy of this ethos, hospitalized individuals are harmed more often than not during the course of their hospital stay.

Historically, infections and other complications were viewed as routine consequences of medical care. For example, 15 to 20 years ago in the neonatal intensive care unit (NICU), bloodstream infections were not uncommon, and many clinicians were not prepared to take ownership for this potentially life-threatening complication. "He or she's 25 weeks" or "he or she's just very sick" were considered plausible explanations for the infant's medical complication. Hospitalized individuals *are* more vulnerable and susceptible to bloodstream infections and a whole host of other hospital-related complications and adverse events. It is this intrinsic vulnerability that demands health care professionals demonstrate prudence, caution, and compassion with every patient interaction. It is incumbent on the health care team to "First do no harm."

The challenge in minimizing the risk of harm to the hospitalized health care consumer is in understanding what constitutes harm—is it physical, emotional, or both? Are there acceptable inherent risks associated with hospitalization? What are the contributing factors?

What Constitutes Medical Harm?

The term medical harm was first coined in 1991 in the benchmark study published in the *New England Journal of Medicine* looking at the incidence of adverse events and negligence in hospitalized patients. The study concluded that there was a substantial amount of injury from medical management in hospitalized individuals and that many of these injuries were the result of substandard care (Brennan et al., 1991).

Adverse events pose a heavy burden on the patient, family, and health care delivery system. A decade following this study the health care industry continues to struggle to deliver safe quality care. Frequently cited adverse events (or preventable medical harm) by The Joint Commission, Centers for Medicare and Medicaid Services (CMS), and other quality health care agencies include pressure ulcers, patient falls, catheter-associated urinary tract infection, central line–associated bloodstream infections, ventilator-associated pneumonia, and surgical site infections. With the exception of suicide risk assessment and prevention, little attention is paid to the emotional, psychosocial, and mental health outcomes associated with hospitalization.

Davydow, Katon, and Zatzick (2009) present a review of the literature, looking at the psychiatric morbidity and functional impairment of survivors of burns, traumatic injuries, and ICU stays for other critical illnesses. The evidence substantiates a significant risk of emotional and psychosocial impairment as a consequence of hospitalization across these three diagnostic domains. In a subsequent publication, Davydow, Richardson, Zatzick, and Katon (2010) looked at the psychiatric morbidity in pediatric ICU survivors and concluded that there is significant compromise to the mental well-being of pediatric ICU survivors related to their hospitalization. Maroney (2003) presents a thoughtful and comprehensive review on the potential effects of stress and trauma associated with hospitalization on premature infants and their impact on long-term psychoemotional health. The pervasive nature of compromised mental health outcomes across a diverse range of patient populations strongly suggests these findings reveal an additional burden incurred from medical care. As both Maroney (2003) and Davydow et al. (2009, 2010) put forth, clinician caregiving, service delivery characteristics, and the patient's experience of care appear to play a critical role in this form of medical harm.

Inherent Risks of Hospitalization

Certainly, there are no guarantees in health care. Complications arise that cannot be foreseen. Variability in patient responsiveness to treatment strategies and other medical interventions are the inherent risks of hospitalization. "First do no harm" is aimed at mitigating and indeed eliminating preventable medical error and harm to the patient. About 100,000 patients die each year from preventable medical error; an additional 100,000 patients die annually from hospital-acquired infections in the United States.

The majority of health care professionals approach each patient encounter thoughtfully, armed with an existing knowledge base aimed at delivering the best care possible. The challenge to eliminate error and harm is twofold. First, at the individual level, is the existing knowledge base reflective of the latest evidence-based best practices, or is care delivery based on rituals and routines that have been in place for the past 30 years? Second, at the system level, is there a commitment to excellence and a culture of accountability with clearly communicated performance expectations? There is an increasingly popular trend to compare performance and outcomes to neighboring hospitals and national databases.

This focus on mediocrity or being a few points better than another facility falls short of meeting the quality and safety needs of the patients we serve.

Preventable, disease-independent adverse outcomes must be eliminated from the patient's experience of care. Current, evidence-based best practices regarding the procedural elements of care as well as the human aspects of caring must be adopted and integrated into the culture of care—*first do no harm*.

Contributing Factors

Human factors, including the cultural and systemic aspects of the environment of care, play a fundamental role in safety. Health care clinicians in the NICU are faced with a myriad of competing priorities and life-and-death situations. Perceptions about time constraints and a paucity of accountability at the individual and systems levels set the stage for deviations from best-practice standards. Let us consider this sample situation:

> *I observed two nurses working with a baby who was a new admission. There was a contact precaution sign posted on the foot of the warming table. One nurse was wearing gloves, the other nurse was not. I asked a colleague about the contact precautions and was informed that all new admissions were placed on contact precautions until they ruled out for methicillin-resistant* Staphylococcus aureus *(MRSA). Given this information, both nurses should have been wearing gloves during the care interaction with the infant. I left this patient's bedside and moved about the rest of the NICU only to circle back to see if the second nurse had donned her gloves. The scene was as I had left it, one nurse wearing gloves and the other not.*

The risk of not wearing gloves far outweighs any perceived benefit. In not complying with contact precautions protocol, the nurse jeopardized the safety of the infant, herself, and potentially other infants in the NICU. However, this nurse is not singularly culpable for the incorrect practice; her colleague missed an opportunity to redirect the noncompliant nurse.

Depending on the relationship between the two nurses, the compliant nurse may have felt there was too much personal risk in confronting her colleague about her noncompliant behavior, especially when the motive may have been a good one—to render immediate assistance. Maybe the noncompliant nurse does not take feedback well; maybe she is intimidating. Regardless of motive and regardless of personality attributes, in choosing not to comply with the best-practice protocol, the quality and safety of the patient's care were undermined. These types of situations happen far too often in the hospital setting. The Joint Commission issued a sentinel event in 2008 addressing behaviors that undermine a culture of safety.

> Intimidating and disruptive behaviors can foster medical errors, contribute to poor patient satisfaction and to preventable adverse outcomes, increase the cost of care, and cause qualified clinicians, administrators and managers to seek new positions and more professional environments. Safety and quality of patient care is dependent on teamwork, communication, and a collaborative work environment. (The Joint Commission, 2008, p. 1)

The human factor in quality and safety is a key contributor in the mitigation and management of risk. Care team vitality and capacity to communicate, collaborate, and, yes, have crucial conversations with colleagues are quintessential to ensure patient safety.

Never impose on others what you would not choose for yourself.—Confucius

NATIONAL PATIENT SAFETY GOALS IN THE NICU

The National Patient Safety Goals (NPSGs) program was established in 2002 in response to increasing mortality associated with breaches in safety. These goals are developed by a multidisciplinary panel of widely recognized patient safety experts and are comprised of nurses, physicians, pharmacists, risk managers, clinical engineers, and other professionals who have hands-on experience in patient safety issues. A copy of the most recent hospital NPSG list can be found at www.jointcommission.org/standards_information/npsgs.aspx.

The NPSGs include accurate patient identification, improved staff communication, safe use of medications, infection prevention, suicide risk assessment, and prevention of surgical mistakes. For the past decade, infection prevention has been listed as an NPSG. The number-one intervention that can reduce a patient's risk of hospital-acquired infection is adherence to hand hygiene protocol. Despite this very simple strategy, hospitals struggle with compliance to hand hygiene practices. McGuckin, Waterman, and Govednik (2009) completed a 12-month, multicenter collaboration in the United States assessing hand hygiene compliance; their baseline compliance data was 26% for ICUs and 36% for non-ICUs.

Raju, Suresh, and Higgins (2011) present an executive summary of a collaborative workshop organized by the Eunice Kennedy Shriver National Institute of Child Health and Human Development (NICHD). The aim of this workshop was to uncover knowledge gaps and formulate a research and educational agenda looking at patient safety in the context of the NICU. Specific safety topics discussed included resuscitation errors, mechanical ventilation, and the performance of invasive procedures as well as medication errors (including errors in milk feeding), diagnostic errors, and patient misidentification.

The identified knowledge gaps emphasize human factors in care delivery in the NICU.

Adherence to evidence-based best practices in quality and safety is a *caring* action. As outlined in the core measures for age-appropriate care (formerly developmental care), the healing environment core measure set is comprised of the physical, human, and systems attributes (Table 1.1).

Table 1.1 *The Healing Environment*

Attribute	Criteria
A quiet, dimly lit, private environment that promotes safety and sleep	1. Continuous background sound and transient sound in the neonatal intensive care unit (NICU) shall not exceed an hourly continuous noise level (Leq) of 45 decibels (dB) and an hourly L10 (the noise level exceeded for 10% of the time) of 50 dB. Transient sounds or L_{max} (the single highest sound level) shall not exceed 65 dB 2. Ambient light levels ranging from 10–600 lux and 1–60 foot candles shall be adjustable and measured at each infant bed space 3. Physical and auditory privacy is afforded at each patient bed space
A collaborative health care team that emanates teamwork, mindfulness, and caring	1. Interdisciplinary care rounds occur at least weekly 2. Direct care providers demonstrate caring behaviors that include adherence to hand hygiene protocols, cultural sensitivity, open listening skills, and a sensitive relationship orientation 3. Nurse–physician collaboration is defined, practiced, and reinforced on a daily basis
Evidence-based policies, procedures, and resources are available to sustain the healing environment over time	1. Core measures of developmental care provide the standard of care for all patient care providers 2. Resources to support the implementation of developmental care as defined by the core measures are always available 3. A system for staff accountability in the practice of developmental care as outlined by the core measures is operational

Source: Coughlin, Gibbins, and Hoath (2009).

Adoption and integration of evidence-based best practices combined with a culture of accountability result in enhanced patient safety and quality caring. The core measures for age-appropriate care will be presented and discussed in great detail in this book and reflect evidence-based best practices in the care of the premature and critically ill infant hospitalized in the NICU.

THE FUTURE OF HEALTH CARE IN THE NICU

The future of health care is about prevention; prevention not only aimed at physical health but mental health as well. Maureen Bisognano, chief executive officer of the Institute for Healthcare Improvement, presented the keynote address at the 2011 International Forum on Quality and Safety in Health Care (Amsterdam, The Netherlands). Her opening remarks talked about a global imperative aimed at disease prevention and health maintenance. She described the first 5 years of life as basically a gestational period for an individual's health trajectory and that health and wellness begin with healthy choices and habits established in early childhood. As a neonatal clinician this truth resonated with me. I thought about the hospitalized premature and critically ill infants in the NICU and how by simply applying evidence-based best practices in human caring, the health and wellness of this vulnerable population could be positively impacted over their life span. Prevention strategies applied in the NICU not only impact the short-term hospital outcomes but also reduce the burden of disease associated with prematurity and neonatal critical illness.

Premature birth is the leading global cause of death in the newborn period; survivors are highly vulnerable and susceptible to a host of complications with lifelong implications that are reflected in terms of the burden of disease associated with neonatal critical illness. Disability-adjusted life year (DALY) is the metric used to quantify the burden of disease. One DALY represents 1 lost year of a healthy life. The worldwide DALY associated with the perinatal conditions is presented in Figure 1.1.

In trying to dissect these long-term conditions that compromise the quality of life of these individuals, research is pointing to mental illness. Nosarti et al. (2012) investigated the relationship between gestational age and psychiatric disorders in young adult life and discovered that preterm birth was significantly associated with an increased risk of psychiatric hospitalization as an adult. At 20 years of age, former premature very

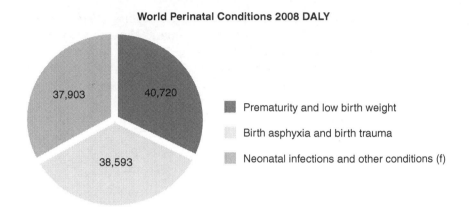

World Perinatal Conditions 2008 DALY

- Prematurity and low birth weight
- Birth asphyxia and birth trauma
- Neonatal infections and other conditions (f)

Figure 1.1 *Most recent data from the World Health Organization global burden of disease summary.*

f = severe neonatal infections and other noninfectious causes arising in the perinatal period.

low birth weight (VLBW) infants and former term infants born small for gestational age (SGA) self-reported compromise to mental well-being, quality of life, and social relations factors when compared to healthy control subjects (Lund et al., 2012). Vanderbilt and Gleason (2010), in an overview of mental health outcomes associated with prematurity, highlight the influence of parental mental wellness in addition to neonatal critical illness as a crucial confounding factor. Although these independent variables are linked to compromised mental health, the combination can lead to significant impairment in long-term neurobehavioral health for the infant. Internalizing behaviors, externalizing behaviors, attention deficit hyperactivity disorder, in addition to more significant psychological pathology, have been described in individuals with a history of neonatal critical illness requiring intensive care treatment.

> *A woman approached me during a break in a learning session I was conducting on trauma-informed care in the NICU. She shared that since childhood she's had a history of terrifying nightmares of people sticking knives into the bottoms of her feet. She described her ritual to protect her feet before she would go to sleep at night, wrapping them up in the blanket for protection; also, when she would have a pedicure she informed me that she had to consciously calm herself and reassure herself that this was not a painful treatment. When the woman took a nursing position in the NICU, she learned about heel sticks (a common method to obtain blood samples from hospitalized infants). She wondered if she had been a*

patient in the NICU and if this was the explanation for her nightmares. When she questioned her mother, she was reassured that she was not in the NICU but did have hyperbilirubinemia as a newborn and that every 4 hours over the course of 2 days she was taken from her mother and brought to the nursery for a heel stick blood sample. The mother revealed that she wanted to accompany her infant daughter, but was told that was not possible and that her infant would be returned quickly. When the baby did return to her mother, she was hysterical, crying, and needed much soothing and consoling from her mother to return to a calm state.

This simple story reflects the 48 hours experience of a relatively healthy individual who was clearly traumatized by her medical experience as a newborn. How many other untold stories from former NICU graduates are linked to nightmares, night terrors, or worse? It is in understanding the impact of complex developmental trauma that neonatal clinicians can better understand the risk associated with NICU hospitalization in this incredibly vulnerable patient population.

The global burden of disease associated with mental illness has profound individual and socioeconomic implications. The majority of mental disorders present themselves in early childhood and/or adolescents. The *Diagnostic and Statistical Manual of Mental Disorders* published by the American Psychiatric Association provides standard criteria for the classification of various mental disorders. Using this reference manual, the World Health Organization (WHO, 2008, 2013), in an update from world mental health surveys, provides information about lifetime prevalence estimates of various psychological pathologies around the world (Figure 1.2). Interestingly, anxiety disorders are consistently found to be the most prevalent class of mental disorders in the population, affecting 31% of the population in the United States (13.85% worldwide; Kessler et al., 2009). Despite the prevalence of anxiety disorders, they are often underrecognized and undertreated when presented in the primary care setting. Several classifications of anxiety disorders include generalized anxiety disorder, panic disorder, acute stress disorder, and posttraumatic stress disorder. In understanding that hospitalization in the NICU is a traumatic life event, clinicians are better prepared to incorporate evidence-based best practices to minimize and mitigate the associated toxic stress and favorably impact long-term mental health outcomes.

The enormity of this problem worldwide compels the global health care community to investigate and operationalize evidence-based best caring strategies aimed at the preservation of mental wellness

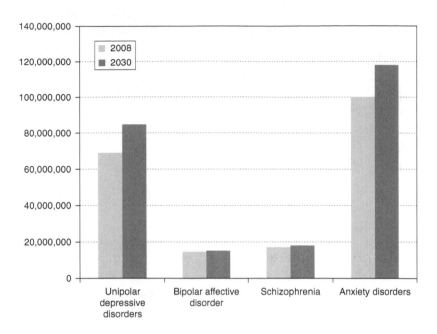

Figure 1.2 *Global DALY of neuropsychiatric conditions adapted from WHO global burden of disease summary.*

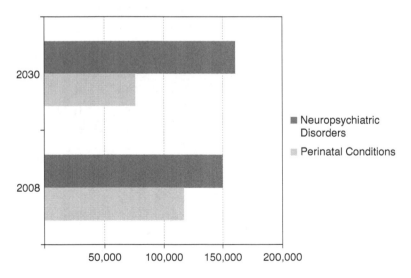

Figure 1.3 *Comparison of perinatal and neuropsychiatric conditions from WHO GBD summary.* ⁓ ·

GBD, global burden of disease.

and prevention of psychological pathologies associated with early life trauma.

Despite projected decreases in global DALY associated with perinatal conditions, the burden of disease associated with neuropsychiatric disorders is increasing. Are we seeing an increase in these psychological pathologies in the setting of improved survival rates in extremely premature and critically ill infants (Figure 1.3)?

Trauma-informed age-appropriate care emulates the moral imperative of "first do no harm" and is a first step in reducing the long-term sequelae associated with NICU hospitalization.

> *Through this approach critically ill preterm infants are treated as we ourselves would hope to be treated in similar situations.*—Maureen Hack

CHAPTER 2: *Vulnerability of the Premature and Hospitalized Infant*

Neonates of all gestational ages share similar vulnerabilities across physiologic, neurobiologic, and psychoemotional domains. The severity of the implications of these vulnerabilities may vary based on underlying disease processes as well as environmental and experiential influences during hospitalization and the postdischarge milieu.

This chapter will outline the age-specific needs of the premature and critically ill, hospitalized infant across physiologic, neurobiologic, and psychoemotional domains. Alterations in meeting these age-appropriate needs associated with acute care hospitalization and life-threatening illness are depicted as developmental trauma. Consequences of developmental trauma are presented from the literature across these same domains and provide a better understanding of how the delivery of trauma-informed age-appropriate care in the neonatal intensive care unit (NICU) can and should be modified to mitigate these deleterious outcomes.

AGE-SPECIFIC NEEDS OF THE PREMATURE AND HOSPITALIZED INFANT

Understanding the developmental requisites for successful human transformation from neonate to adult is crucial for the neonatal clinician. The age-specific needs of the premature and hospitalized infant are disease independent and reflect human developmental essentials. Developmental biology and the research on epigenetic influences coupled with growing literature in the field of developmental psychology present neonatal clinicians with a rich body of knowledge aimed at transforming caring interactions to promote optimal growth and development.

Physiologic Needs

> *Effects vary with the conditions which bring them to pass, but laws do not vary. Physiological and pathological states are ruled by the same forces; they differ only because of the special conditions under which the vital laws manifest themselves.*—Claude Bernard

Unlike many of our mammalian counterparts, humans are born dependent on adult caregivers to meet physiologic needs for survival. Maslow's hierarchy of needs places these physiologic requisites at the base of his pyramid, which includes food, water, air, sleep, homeostasis, and excretion. The physiologic needs of the premature and critically ill neonate are complex and complicated by underlying pathologic processes and systemic mechanisms that attempt to maintain homeostasis.

The stress response attempts to restore homeostasis and is successful when the individual is able to adapt to the stressor and re-establish equilibrium. Stressors that assault this fragile patient population extend beyond their primary diagnosis and include maternal separation, pain, isolation, sleep deprivation, and other environmental and experiential events that activate the hypothalamic–pituitary–adrenal (HPA) axis.

The allostatic mechanism responds to stressors by increasing circulating catecholamines and glucocorticoids to prepare the organism for "fight or flight." When the stress experience is prolonged and there is a paucity of consistent and effective interventions to ameliorate or mitigate the situation, the stress becomes toxic and is described as an allostatic load. Toxic stress is the prolonged activation of the HPA axis and autonomic nervous system, which can disrupt brain architecture and other organ systems as well as increase the risk for stress-related disease processes and cognitive impairment. Maslow's physiologic fundamentals take on crucial significance for these fragile individuals in this setting.

Cardiopulmonary function must ensure adequate gas exchange and sufficient tissue perfusion to preserve systemic cellular integrity and end-organ survival. Metabolic operations must provide sufficient substrates for cellular activity. The role of the endocrine system along with the central nervous system responds to and directs integrative functions responsive to both internal and external environmental influences.

A review of each body system's contribution to survival is beyond the scope of this book; however, an appreciation of the dynamic nature of physiologic function is requisite for the neonatal nurse. Nutrition, hydration, thermal neutrality, pain management, and the protection of sleep create a life-sustaining backdrop to physiologic integrity of the medically compromised infant. These quintessential elements provide much needed energy to support and promote healing, growth, and development for these vulnerable individuals.

Calculating energy expenditure for the critically ill infant is a challenge at best. Most neonatal dieticians focus on maintaining (or strive to achieve) fetal growth rates. The best measure for success in meeting the metabolic demands of this fragile population is linear growth. Although weight gain can be a supportive variable in assessing overall growth, it is in the ability to lay down new tissue reflected in linear growth that the nutritional intervention can be deemed successful. That being said, promoting growth is not only about nutrition; the caring NICU clinician must be able to identify activities that compound the infant's caloric needs and manage and minimize this excessive expenditure. Activities that exacerbate the energy demands of the premature and critically ill infant are associated with activation of the stress response mechanism and include (but are not limited to) excessive noise and light, abrupt care encounters, undermanaged pain and stress, family separation, and sleep deprivation.

Moore, Berger, and Wilson (2012) put forth a proposed model linking complications of prematurity with allostasis, allostatic load, and associated physiologic response patterns (both adaptive and maladaptive). In a recent review article by Cuesta and Singer (2012), the authors link critical illness with a "stress-related decompensation syndrome." Understanding the link between physiologic stability and environmental and experiential stressors is crucial for neonatal clinicians.

Neurobiological Needs

Experience can become biology.—Dr. Bruce Perry

The brain is a living, social structure that demands stimulation through human interaction, nurturance, and attachment. In the absence of social support and interactivity, young humans fail to thrive. Renee Spitz published his observations of infants and young children cared for in an orphanage in 1951 and coined the term "hospitalism" as the condition these infants acquired as a result of emotional deprivation. The infants he observed received custodial care during critical stages of development; however, despite meeting the fundamental physiologic needs of these infants, they went on to suffer profound neurodevelopmental consequences from their experiences. Spitz described in detail the cognitive, behavioral, and motor deficits of these infants. (Review Spitz's clinical observations and conclusions at www.youtube.com/watch?v=VvdOe10vrs4.)

The human brain is comprised of billions of neurons. In fact, a recent estimate of the neuronal density in the adult human brain was placed at 86 billion neurons and approximately 85 billion glial cells, with only 19% of these neurons being located in the cerebral cortex (Azevedo et al., 2009). When you consider that by week 10 of gestation the human fetus is producing on average 250,000 neurons/minute, and the bulk of brain development occurring during this critical stage of development is primarily taking place in the brainstem, cerebellum, and subcortex (the limbic system), it gives one pause to appreciate the critical role these primal neurologic structures play in the life of an individual.

To understand the neurobiological needs of the premature and critically ill, hospitalized infant, one must first understand the dynamics of neurogenesis during critical and sensitive periods of development. Experience-expectant development, usually associated with sensory and perceptual functions, generally is a time-limited event. If the expected experience is altered or absent during the designated critical period, then the corresponding neural networks will be impacted. Experience-dependent development, which occurs at any point along the life cycle, is influenced by individual life experiences (usually within the context of relationship) that adjusts and/or modifies brain architecture and function. Learning is the best example of experience-dependent activity.

The rich sensory environment of the intrauterine world nurtures the dynamic explosion of neuronal and nonneuronal cell proliferation, creating the canvas for the human experience to be interpreted and translated into how the individual will interact with the world. In an ordered developmental sequence beginning in the subcortex, the brainstem and cerebellum organize to regulate involuntary functions such as temperature, heart rate, and basic reflexes. Building on this primal apparatus is the limbic system (primarily the amygdala, hippocampus, hypothalamus, and the olfactory bulb). These structures are involved with emotion, memory, and learning. The cerebral cortex, which develops over the latter part of the third trimester and continues to develop and differentiate through adolescence, organizes sensory, motor, and conscious experiences. Neurons are social by nature through experience-expectant and experience-dependent programming—neurons that fire together, wire together (Hebb, 1949).

Through finely tuned and exquisitely specific neurobiological mechanisms and substrates, the human infant's early life experiences model and shape relational processes that become part of the infant's identity into childhood and beyond (Roisman & Fraley, 2012). These neonatal individuals require early life experiences that support and reinforce neural connections related to security, connectedness, attachment, self-regulation, and love (Esch & Stefano, 2011). Through positive social experiences during critical and sensitive periods of development, neuro-chemical systems establish a lattice of synaptic connections that facilitate the development of resilience and balanced state and emotion regulation (Solodkin & Stern, 2012).

Psychoemotional Needs

Since the earliest period of our life was preverbal, everything depended on emotional interaction. Without someone to reflect our emotions, we had no way of knowing who we were.—John Bradshaw, *Healing the Shame That Binds You*

Erik Erikson's stages of psychosocial development span the life continuum from infancy to adulthood. The first stage of psychosocial development is trust versus mistrust. The life-stage virtue associated with this developmental stage is hope, and the existential question posed is, "Can I trust the world?" The parent figure(s) and/or the primary caregiver represent the world and the answer to this existential question hinges on the relational experiences between infant and caregiver (Tronick & Beeghly, 2011).

The relational experience is attachment. In the original work of John Bowlby, titled *Attachment* (1969), he introduces the concept "that the attachment relationship directly influences the infant's capacity to cope with stress" (Schore, 2001b). The attachment relationship underpins the psychoemotional needs of the neonate. This attachment is founded on trust. To establish trust, the attachment relationship must include bidirectional communication between infant and adult and demonstrate compassion, consistency, and competence with each infant encounter.

Bowlby's proposed theory of attachment focused on species survival as the premise of his construct. In clinical observations of infant–caregiver interactions he and his contemporaries discover that establishing relationships is a primary human instinct and this instinct preserves the continuation of the species. Bowlby suggests that the infant creates an "Internal Working Model" of him- or herself and the caregiver that will frame and guide the infant's behaviors and his or her expectations of the caregiver. What the infant is looking for is a consistent and reliable sense of security—a security that is perceived and registered on a neurobiological and a psychoemotional level.

Relationships impact biology and are mediated by emotions. The first and formative relationship for humans is with mother, in utero. The fetus hears the mother's voice, experiences fluctuations in the maternal cardiovascular responsiveness to extrauterine stimuli, and is primed by the maternal mood and emotional integrity. The internal milieu of the healthy intrauterine world conveys safety, love, and predictability, which enable the fetus to develop according to his or her genetic script. In the setting of a compromised intrauterine environment (maternal medical conditions, mental illness, or toxic substance exposure), placental function may be impaired and become the object for epigenetic dysregulation or changes in gene expression that are not actually encoded in DNA but are modified by environmental and experiential events.

NICU admission as a traumatic event in the life of the infant marks an abrupt and protracted separation from mother superimposed by life-threatening illness and all the associated medical interventions and invasive procedures. Regardless of the infant's diagnostic condition, the primal needs of the newborn (proximity to his or her mother, predictability of comfort, safety, and nurturance) are crucial for optimal psychoemotional outcomes, physical health, and recovery from the trauma associated with neonatal intensive care.

Through consistent, compassionate social support including parental proximity, caregiver presence, and the implementation of age-appropriate care strategies, stress and distress associated with the NICU experience are effectively managed to minimize long-term psychoemotional adverse outcomes.

TRAUMA AND THE PREMATURE AND HOSPITALIZED INFANT

A traumatic event is an experience that causes physical, emotional, psychological distress, or harm. It is an event that is perceived and experienced as a threat to one's safety or to the stability of one's world.—www.nlm.nih.gov/medlineplus/ency/article/001924.htm

Developmental trauma is a traumatic event that occurs during a sensitive and critical period of growth and maturation for the neonate. Hospitalization in a NICU is an example of a very complex developmental trauma to the infant as well as the parents and the family as a whole.

This author recognizes the parental trauma associated with this experience and defers and refers the reader to the myriad of experts who have contributed to our understanding of the trauma experience of the NICU parent. This book focuses on the trauma experience of the infant. That being said, the parental trauma experience will impact the infant by way of the parent figures' capacity to attach and establish a base of security for the infant, not only during the hospital experience but also in the post-NICU discharge period.

Emotional and social deprivation during critical periods of development have been linked with lifelong consequences across physical, neurobiological, and psychoemotional domains. In addition, experiences with stress and pain that are either unmanaged or undermanaged and sleep deprivation add an additional allostatic load that compromises the infant's biological integrity and undermines maturation, growth, and recovery.

The quality of the relationship infants have with their caregivers plays a critical role in regulating the infant's stress response. Relationships that convey safety, security, and love cultivate resilience (Wu et al., 2013).

CONSEQUENCES OF UNRESOLVED TRAUMA

Environments designed to care for neonatal individuals must recognize and provide for the age-appropriate needs of this incredibly fragile and susceptible patient population. When these needs are met consistently and reliably, the infant develops resilience and is better prepared to manage stressful encounters over the course of his or her life. If these needs are not met, the infant will experience lifelong consequences associated with the toxic stress of the NICU milieu and all of the associated ramifications linked with physiologic, neurobiologic, and psychoemotional domains (Chu & Lieberman, 2010; Pechtel & Pizzagalli, 2011).

Physiologic Consequences

Prematurity and critical illness during the neonatal period expose the developing human to excessive stressors that influence and alter physiologic and homeostatic mechanisms and have lifelong implications for the affected individual. In addition, pathophysiologic sequelae associated with the various medical conditions warranting NICU hospitalization can confound the individual's ability to self-regulate and establish a secure base with an attachment figure. Traumatic experiences occurring during sensitive and vulnerable periods of development have been specifically linked with immune reactivity and altered HPA axis performance.

Simple routine care delivery in the NICU precipitates major fluctuations in cerebral hemodynamics (Limperopoulos et al., 2008). These routine cares include minor manipulations, diaper changes, endotracheal tube (ETT) suctioning, ETT repositioning, and other more complex care events. Fluctuations in cerebral perfusion have been associated with parenchymal brain injury and long-term neurodevelopmental outcomes. In addition to cerebral hemodynamics, there are a variety of care interactivities that are known to elicit a pain response in the hospitalized neonate and yet go unmanaged or undermanaged. The literature is replete with research on the neonatal pain experience and the long-term implications of undertreated pain (Bouza, 2009; Grunau, 2002; Grunau, Holsti, & Peters, 2006). Effective evidence-based care strategies are available to mitigate and manage these painful events. Feeding tube placement has been associated with measurable increases in biobehavioral pain responses (using the Premature Infant Pain Profile [PIPP]; Kristoffersen, Skogvoll, & Hafström, 2011). Diaper change and bathing have been documented as stressful events for the hospitalized infant (Comaru & Miura, 2009; Liaw, Yang, Chou, Yang, & Chao, 2010; Liaw, Yang, Yuh, & Yin, 2006; Mörelius, Hellström-Westas, Carlén, Norman, & Nelson, 2006). The lifelong implications of excessive and, yes, toxic stress are well reported in the literature. HPA axis dysfunction (a consequence of toxic stress) has been an associated precursor to insulin resistance, autoimmune disorders of the gut, regional alterations in brain structure and function, as well as growth failure (Brame & Singer, 2010; Johnson & Gunner, 2011; Konturek, Brzozowski, & Konturek, 2011; Kristoffersen et al., 2011; Smith et al., 2011; Srinivasan, 2012).

The role of oxidative stress in the perinatal origins of adult disease is an emerging pathogenic component (Davidge, Morton, & Rueda-Clausen, 2008). Oxidative stress is an imbalance between the production of oxygen-free radicals (often associated with hypoxic/ischemic conditions) and available antioxidants that scavenge these metabolites that are toxic to the surrounding cellular environment (Durackova, 2010). Procedural pain has been elegantly described as a precursor to oxidative stress in premature infants (Slater et al., 2012); the oxygen-free radicals produced during procedural pain can induce an apoptosis and even damage DNA structures. Increases in oxidative stress biomarkers have been associated with necrotizing enterocolitis and perinatal brain injury (Moore et al., 2012; Perrone et al., 2012; Taylor, Edwards, & Mehmet, 1999).

An additional physiologic stressor with long-term adverse consequences is sleep deprivation. The sleep needs of the premature and hospitalized infant range between 17 and 22 hours per day. Adequate sleep during the neonatal period is linked with linear growth, synaptogenesis, memory, learning, and immune function (Graven & Browne, 2008b; Imeri & Opp, 2009; Lampl & Johnson, 2011; Peirano & Algarin, 2007; Peirano, Algarín, & Uauy, 2003).

The physiologic consequences of stress are mediated at the level of the central nervous system by way of the HPA axis. In response to a stressor there is a surge in circulating catecholamines and cortisol to activate the fight or flight response, which includes circulatory changes, to redirect blood flow and enhance cardiovascular tone to meet the needed energy demands of vital organs during an acute event. When the stress is unrelenting and becomes a chronic situation, the hormonal environment becomes toxic to developing neurons and other vulnerable organ systems (renal, gastrointestinal [GI], cardiopulmonary, endocrine, and immune systems). Prolonged activation of the stress response increases the risk of cognitive dysfunction, cardiovascular disease, diabetes, and mental health challenges (Lai & Huang, 2011).

Developmental trauma is cultivated in an environment of toxic stress or an inability of the normal stress response to restore homeostatic control and facilitate adaptation (Rifkin-Graboi et al., 2009). For infants, this occurs in the absence of an intervening adult mediator of the experience. Stress is a reality in the neonatal ICU, but failure to manage the infant's experience through authentic presence, thoughtful procedural care delivery, protecting and promoting sleep, engaging and empowering parenting, and effectively managing painful and stressful events yields lifelong physiologic consequences.

In a 2012 policy statement, the American Academy of Pediatrics (AAP) states,

> AAP is committed to leveraging science to inform the development of innovative strategies to reduce the precipitants of toxic stress in young children and to mitigate their negative effects

on the course of development and health across the life span. (Committee on Psychosocial Aspects of Child, 2012).

Neurobiological Consequences

At a neurobiological level, the early life experience of the premature and critically ill, hospitalized infant becomes a blueprint for future interactions with stress as well as designing the platform for how these individuals relate in the world. The neuroendocrine and neuroimmune systems are programmed by the hormonal milieu of the brain mediated by the HPA axis, specifically catecholamines and cortisol. In the absence of age-appropriate nurturing care experiences, the developing brain is exposed to hyperactivation of the HPA axis and a resetting of the stress response occurs. This reset is in the way of either a hyperresponsive (fight/aggression) or hyporesponsive (fright/withdrawal) behavior pattern.

Maternal separation has been documented as the primary stressor for neonates, and Lajud, Roque, Cajero, Gutiérrez-Ospina, and Torner (2012) demonstrated that this early life stressor decreases hippocampal neurogenesis, and alters HPA axis function and the coping capacity in these individuals as adults. Deprived early life experiences have also been associated with anxiety and depression-like behaviors and increases in aggression linked to altered oxytocin immunoreactivity in the paraventricular nucleus located in the hypothalamus (Veenema, 2012).

Repetitive and chronic pain experiences trigger a hyperinnervation of the pain system, which can lower pain thresholds and even create a hypersensitivity to nonpainful stimulation (like handling or touch). These persistent pain experiences change the molecular structure of the brain and are hardwired into the hippocampus as subconscious memory (Brummelte et al., 2012). These memories can surface in later life as somatic illness such as fibromyalgia, chronic pain syndrome, and other types of conditions that elude diagnosis (Low & Schweinhardt, 2012).

The oxytocin molecule has been linked to the regulation of a variety of behaviors related to social interactions, parturition and lactation, attachment, feeding, learning, and pain perception. Oxytocin has been described as the antithesis to cortisol. Where cortisol is associated with the fight or flight/fright response, oxytocin is the calming and connectedness hormone. Activities that release oxytocin in the neonate include suckling, skin-to-skin contact, nonthreatening physical and tactile stimulation, as well as social vocalizations (Seltzer, Ziegler, & Pollak, 2010).

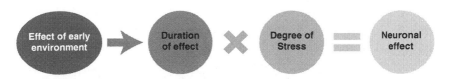

Figure 2.1 *The influence of early life experiences is contingent on the duration of the experience and the degree of stress (mild, moderate, or toxic).*

In the setting of toxic stress and developmental trauma, oxytocin has been demonstrated to limit HPA hyperactivity (Carter, 2003; Yeğen, 2010). Oxytocin has potent antistress properties but is only available when stimulated for release. In addition, oxytocin has anti-inflammatory properties that operate at various levels of the inflammatory process. Hence, if secretion were stimulated routinely, many of the systemic and neuronal complications could be minimized. This outcome is only possible in the setting of interventions that stimulate the release of oxytocin. Similar reports are seen with regard to oxytocin and its antinociceptive properties, which have been demonstrated in clinical observations of the benefit of breast-feeding and skin-to-skin care for premature and hospitalized newborns as a treatment intervention to manage pain associated with heel stick.

Sustained exposure to early life stressors alters functional orientation of the HPA axis as well as limbic structures (primarily the amygdala and hippocampus; Lai & Huang, 2011; Figure 2.1).

Stress is a daily encounter in the NICU. Exposure to stress creates opportunities for adaptation when moderated and managed effectively. In the absence of consistent interventions to manage and mitigate the stress and distress associated with the NICU experience, these tiny individuals are at increased risk for mental illness (National Scientific Council on the Developing Child, 2005).

Psychoemotional Consequences

In the setting of events that deviate from the genetically programmed experiential expectations of the neonate, adverse psychoemotional sequelae follow. Maternal separation is the number-one stressor in neonates, and when this is combined with an environment of care that is inconsistent and unpredictable, the infant is unable to effectively adapt to his or her situation.

René Spitz observed that infants hospitalized in environments that attended solely to basic custodial needs induced an "anaclitic depression" in the observed infants (Spitz, 1945, 1951). Additional work by Spitz's contemporaries made similar observations of institutionalized infants that lay the foundation of our understanding today of the devastating effect of maternal separation and relational isolation. Goldfarb (1945) described features of the environments that produced these behavioral manifestations in infants, including (a) an absence of age-appropriate stimulation, (b) a paucity of psychological interactions and reciprocal relationships with adult caregivers, and (c) an absence of normal identification of self (we define who we are in relation to other; Tronick & Beeghly, 2011).

Social isolation has profound implications for long-term psychoemotional health and well-being. Wired for survival, the rhesus monkey experiments of Harry Harlow (1958) and Harlow and Zimmermann (1959) highlight profound adaptation to adverse circumstances at a psychoemotional price—aberrant attachment. Please take a moment to view a video of Harlow's study on dependency in monkeys at this link: www.youtube.com/watch?v=OrNBEhzjg8I.

John Bowlby's theory of attachment, validated by the work of Mary Ainsworth, revolutionized our understanding of profound importance and lifelong implications of the infant–parent relationship. Disturbances in this relationship, particularly during the first 3 months of life, through separation not only influence the life experience of the infant but also establish an internal working model of relationships across the infant's life span, mental wellness, and psychoemotional stability (Bretherton, 1992).

The attachment relationship has a direct impact on an individual's capacity for emotion regulation. Emotion regulation is an individual's ability to respond to a situation or circumstances in an effective way. The psychoemotional consequences of developmental trauma during the neonatal period manifest in the infant's emotion regulatory skill set (Calkins & Hill, 2007). NICU clinicians must understand how stressors in the NICU are mediated by attachment-related strategies linked to emotions; if the attachment is not secure or is inconsistent and unstable, an emotional response pattern is cultivated and predicated on the attachment experience which then becomes the individual's default emotional response to stressful circumstances beyond the NICU. These emotional response patterns may be maladaptive to the situation and, if they persist, disrupt other processes necessary for social relations and a functional social existence (Cole, Michel, & Teti, 1994).

SUMMARY

Premature infants and critically ill newborns are extremely vulnerable and susceptible to altered development across physical, neurobiological, and psychoemotional domains. Recognizing the age-appropriate needs of this very special population and understanding the consequences of not meeting these vital requisites compel the caring neonatal clinician to modify the care experience of these individuals consistently and reliably.

CHAPTER 3: *Trauma-Informed Age-Appropriate Care*

WHAT IS TRAUMA-INFORMED AGE-APPROPRIATE CARE?

Trauma-informed age-appropriate care is a developmental concept that recognizes the physiological, neurobiological, and psychoemotional sequelae of trauma in early life and aims to mitigate the deleterious effects associated with the trauma experience through the provision of evidence-based, age-appropriate caring strategies.

Trauma-Informed Care

The concept of trauma-informed care has its origins in the field of behavioral health. The National Child Traumatic Stress Network (NCTSN) was established in 2000 as part of the Children's Health Act funded by the Substance Abuse and Mental Health Services Administration (SAMHSA). The mission of the NCTSN is to develop treatment and intervention strategies, provide training, and design system changes that integrate trauma-informed evidence-based practices in all child-serving systems.

The NCTSN has created a "Pediatric Medical Traumatic Stress Toolkit for Health Care Providers" (www.nctsnet.org/trauma-types/pediatric-medical-traumatic-stress-toolkit-for-health-care-providers), which provides clinicians with generalized strategies in managing the trauma experience of the hospitalized child. Although not specifically addressing the neonatal intensive care unit (NICU) experience, the themes and concepts presented in this resource are beneficial for NICU clinicians. The take-home message from the NCTSN is that child traumatic stress is one of the most treatable mental health problems of childhood; receiving timely and appropriate intervention can assist in restoring wellness.

Bringing a trauma perspective to the neonatal intensive care environment is vital to improve short- and long-term outcomes in the premature and critically ill infant population (Grasso et al., 2013). NICU clinicians who view care delivery through a trauma lens are better prepared to support the infant's mental health during the experience of medical trauma associated with hospitalization (Sprenath et al., 2011).

For the premature and critically ill, hospitalized infant, timely and age-appropriate interventions take on new meaning, as the trauma experience is ever present during the hospital stay. Trauma-informed clinicians consistently and reliably manage the toxic stress associated with each and every care interaction and thereby reduce the lifelong implications associated with early life trauma.

Age-Appropriate Care

The Joint Commission (TJC) introduced the term *age-appropriate care* in 1991 with the goal of establishing minimum competencies for individualized, patient-centered care delivery. Recognizing that patient needs and capabilities are different at various stages over the life continuum, mandating competence in age-appropriate care ensures that the patient's experience of care aligns with his or her developmental, biological, psychological, and socioemotional needs.

The provision of age-appropriate care in a hospital setting can be daunting, with competing clinical priorities, pressure of cost containment, maintaining workflow efficiencies, and rigid hospital routines and rituals. Recognizing the patient as person is an imperative in the provision of safe, quality health care.

Parental presence, proximity, protection, and responsiveness to the infant's needs and experiences are the hallmark of neonatal age-appropriate care. In the NICU, these basic needs often fall through the cracks of a technologically oriented, diagnosis-driven, high-paced environment focused on task completion.

Meeting the age-appropriate needs of the premature and critically ill, hospitalized infant demands active participation of the NICU clinician in facilitating infant–parent engagement, role modeling safe infant care practices within the context of the infant's medical liabilities, and participating in the *human dimensions* of the infant–caregiver dyad relationship.

NICU clinicians become an extension of the parents (in their absence) and are interwoven into the infant's social network in the NICU. Neonatal clinicians who are responsive to the age-appropriate needs of their tiny patients are protective; minimize/mitigate distress and pain; and reassure and promote comfort, security, and trust with every infant interaction.

Trauma-Informed Age-Appropriate Care in the NICU

In understanding the biological and developmental needs of the neonate and the negative impact of trauma on these biological and developmental events, NICU clinicians can consciously and consistently manage the premature and critically ill infant's experience of care. This disease-independent approach is mediated by our empathy and acknowledgment of our shared humanity with the hospitalized neonate.

This relational synchrony of the infant–adult dyad (whether parent or clinician) enhances the infant's understanding of his- or herself in relation to the world around him or her communicated through his or her emotional experiences. If the emotional experience is one of indifference, or lack of caring, this translates to a negative experience of self and the world; however, if the emotional experience is of support, comfort, and love, then the infant is encouraged, validated, and develops a positive sense of self and positive perception of the other.

Trauma-informed age-appropriate care in the NICU validates the personhood of the infant, acknowledges the medical trauma experience, and utilizes all available age-appropriate, evidence-based interventions to support the infant. Operationalizing this concept in clinical practice establishes an environment of trust and security for the infant that is fundamental for his or her future physical and mental health and wellness.

THEORETICAL FRAMEWORK FOR TRAUMA-INFORMED AGE-APPROPRIATE CARE IN THE NICU

Developmental psychology, psychiatry, neuroscience, and nursing theory frame the concept of trauma-informed age-appropriate care in the NICU. From the work of developmental psychologist Erik Erikson and developmental psychiatrist Heidelise Als to nurse theorist Myra Levine and neuroscientist Bruce McEwen, neonatal clinicians are compelled to meet the fundamental, interpersonal, holistic human needs of the fragile and vulnerable individuals cared for in the NICU.

Erik Erikson

Hope is both the earliest and the most indispensable virtue inherent in the state of being alive. If life is to be sustained hope must remain, even where confidence is wounded, trust impaired.—Erik Erikson

Erik Erikson's theory of psychosocial development focuses on the development of ego identity and how this identity emerges from our social interactions. Erikson purports that competence motivates behavior and action, and so with each stage of development the individual is challenged to build competency in a stage-specific aspect of psychosocial development. Erikson delineates eight stages of psychosocial development (Figure 3.1) beginning with infancy (age 0–1 year), where the task is the development of trust and a lack of resolution with this task leads to mistrust. Due to an infant's complete dependence on his or her caregiver, the development of trust is determined by the caregiver's capacity to respond to the infant's needs consistently and reliably. Erikson summarizes that if an infant is successful in developing trust, he or she will feel safe and secure in the world; however, if caregivers are inconsistent, emotionally unavailable, or rejecting, the infant will feel abandoned, leading to feelings of fear and a belief that the world is a scary and unsafe place.

Erikson's theory underpins the need for trauma-informed age-appropriate care in the NICU. The NICU experience by definition is a traumatic life event and causes a dramatic interruption in the psychosocial development of the premature and critically ill infant. As neonatal clinicians are interwoven into the social context of the infant's life during the NICU stay, they play a crucial role in whether or not the infant will develop trust and hope. Pain and stress are everyday realities in the NICU; it is

1. HOPE—basic trust versus mistrust (0–1 year)
2. WILL—autonomy versus shame and doubt (1–3 years)
3. PURPOSE—initiative versus guilt (3–6 years)
4. COMPETENCE—industry versus inferiority (6–11 years)
5. FIDELITY—identity versus role confusion (12–mid-20s)
6. LOVE—intimacy versus isolation (young adult—mid-20s to early 40s)
7. CARING—generativity versus stagnation (40s to 60s)
8. WISDOM—ego integrity versus despair (60 years or older)

Figure 3.1 *Erikson's life-stage virtues and psychosocial stages of development.*

in *how* neonatal clinicians predictably and reliably manage these experiences that opportunities to build trusting and secure relationships are created between infant and caregiver that give way to resilience.

Heidelise Als

Human interactive caring work is much harder than any kind of mechanical and technical work. . . . NICU caregivers are expected to be fully engaged and emotionally present and attuned at all times.—Heidelise Als

Heidelise Als, PhD, a pioneer in the work of developmentally supportive care, advanced the knowledge of preterm infant behavior through her Synactive Theory of Development, which proposes, "development proceeds through continuous balancing of approach and avoidance, continuous intraorganism subsystem interaction and differentiation and organism–environment interaction to realize a hierarchical species unique developmental agenda" (Als, 1982).

Grounded by the Synactive Theory, Als, whose early collaboration with T. Berry Brazelton influenced and ignited her passion for the neonatal patient population, developed the Assessment of Preterm Infants' Behavior (APIB) tool. This tool, an adaptation of Dr. Brazelton's Neonatal Behavioral Assessment Scale (NBAS), refined indicators of self-regulatory efforts and thresholds for disorganization based on the preterm infant's subsystems' interactions with the environment. These subsystems include autonomic integrity, motor activity, infant state, attention capacity, and self-regulation (or the ability of the infant to restore stability to self). Infant competence across these five subsystems is communicated as infant biobehavioral cues and informs the NICU clinician about the infant's readiness for a care interaction.

Als went on to develop a training program to be operationalized in the clinical setting to evaluate the tenets of the Synactive Theory and successfully published copiously on the benefits of providing developmentally supportive care to the premature infant patient population. The clinical strategies utilized by Als's training program (Newborn Individualized Developmental Care and Assessment Program [NIDCAP]) resonate with the concept of trauma-informed age-appropriate care in the NICU. Als's framework acknowledges the stress associated with NICU hospitalization, and her assessment criteria provide evidence-based, infant-driven feedback to the neonatal clinician. Understanding the neurodevelopmental competence of the infant is crucial for the trauma-informed clinician, who can then adapt care interactions in response to the infant's subsystem responses.

Myra Levine

> *The nurse enters into a partnership of human experience where sharing moments in time—some trivial, some dramatic—leaves its mark forever on each patient.*—Myra Levine

Myra Estrin Levine completed her Conservational Theory in 1973. This theoretical model focuses on promoting adaptation and maintaining wholeness for the hospitalized individual using principles of conservation. Specifically, Levine describes four conservational principles aimed at preserving the individual's wholeness. These principles are (a) conservation of energy, (b) conservation of structural integrity, (c) conservation of personal integrity, and (d) conservation of social integrity.

In addition to these conservation principles, Levine's model (Figure 3.2) is oriented toward four major concepts: person, environment, nursing, and health. Levine emphasizes the need for congruence between person and environment (both internal environment and external environment) to restore health. The nurse, through human interactions, supports the patient's adaptation to his or her environment while preserving his or her integrity.

Beginning with the external environment, which Levine breaks down into the perceptual, operational, and conceptual components, it becomes apparent how this theory aligns with the concept of a trauma-informed age-appropriate approach to care. The perceptual environment is what the infant responds to through his or her sensory systems. Excessive light and sound cause undue stress on the premature and critically ill infant's physiology; chemical smells and noxious oral/perioral experiences compromise the infant's ability to eat; brusque, poorly supported movements impact fragile vestibular mechanisms and also impact musculoskeletal development; moreover, repeated painful procedures disrupt skin integrity but more importantly alter neural circuitry and undermine the developmental potential of the infant. The operational environment constitutes all forms of radiation, microorganisms, and pollutants, which, in the NICU, includes radiographic exams, risk for nosocomial infection, and other toxins (preservatives and other chemical exposures) associated with medication administration. Lastly,

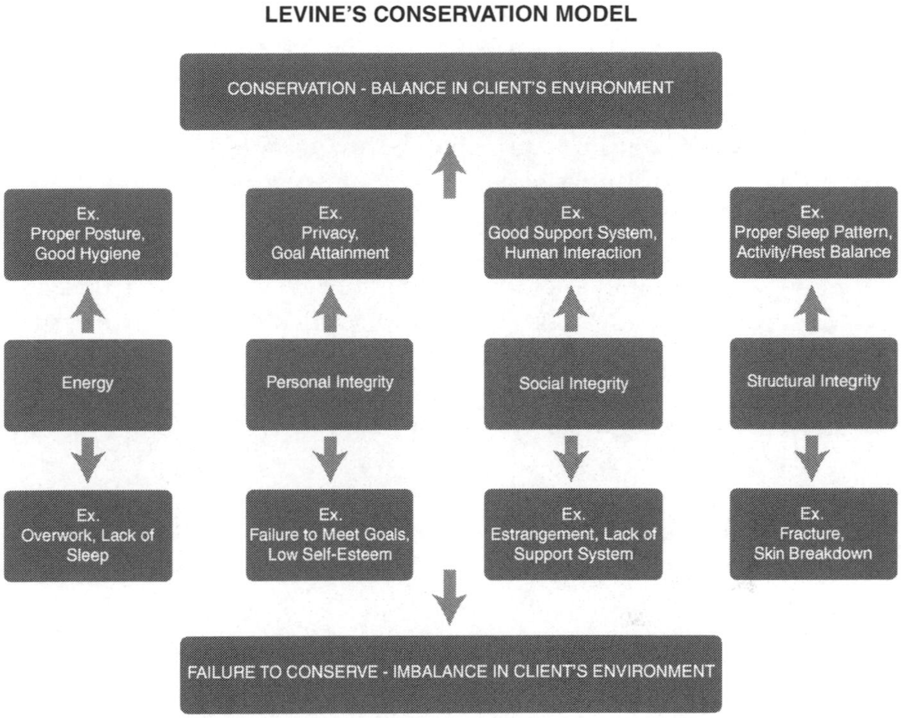

LEVINE'S CONSERVATION MODEL

CONSERVATION - BALANCE IN CLIENT'S ENVIRONMENT

Ex. Proper Posture, Good Hygiene	Ex. Privacy, Goal Attainment	Ex. Good Support System, Human Interaction	Ex. Proper Sleep Pattern, Activity/Rest Balance
Energy	Personal Integrity	Social Integrity	Structural Integrity
Ex. Overwork, Lack of Sleep	Ex. Failure to Meet Goals, Low Self-Esteem	Ex. Estrangement, Lack of Support System	Ex. Fracture, Skin Breakdown

FAILURE TO CONSERVE - IMBALANCE IN CLIENT'S ENVIRONMENT

Figure 3.2 *Levine's conservation model.*

Graph published under Creative Commons license.

the conceptual environment, that aspect of the experience of care which makes up the intangible wholeness of the hospitalized, critically ill infant and includes the exchange of language, emotional experiences and the infant's evolving interpretation of his/her self worth as a human being determined by the experience of care. Collectively, these environmental experiences constitute trauma and require modification and adaptation by the mindful, responsive, trauma-informed clinician.

Bruce McEwen

> *The brain is the key organ of stress processes. It determines what individuals will experience as stressful, it orchestrates how individuals will cope with stressful experiences, and it changes both functionally and structurally as a result of stressful experiences.*—Bruce McEwen

Although Hans Selye was the pioneer of the Stress Response Theory, Bruce McEwen, a noted neuroscientist and neuroendocrinologist, advanced our understanding of the stress response and its mechanisms of action with his extensive study of allostasis and allostatic load. These concepts provide greater insight into the impact of toxic stress on the vulnerable developing brain and physiologic integrity of the hospitalized infant. McEwen elucidates the relationship between homeostasis and allostasis, and describes four types of allodynamic and physiologic responses that undermine restoration of internal equilibrium and reflect allostatic load (Figure 3.3). "These include (a) repeated 'hits' from multiple stressors, (b) a lack of adaptation or habituation, (c) prolonged exposure due to delayed shutdown, and (d) inadequate response that leads to compensatory hyperactivation of other mediators" (McEwen & Gianaros, 2011, pp. 433–434).

McEwen's model clearly aligns with the need for trauma-informed age-appropriate care in the NICU. When reviewing the allodynamic mechanisms within the context of prematurity and critical illness in the

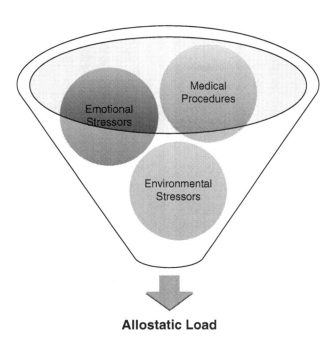

Allostatic Load

Figure 3.3 *Patient experience and allostatic load.*

newborn, these individuals are routinely exposed to multiple, repetitive noxious stressors; due to their immaturity, they have minimal adaptive resources and often shut down through autonomic bailout (cardiopulmonary instability) or dissociation in response to their fight or flight/fight or fright mechanism, and these insufficient response capabilities alter how these individuals are able to handle stress over their life span.

EVIDENCE THAT SUPPORTS TRAUMA-INFORMED AGE-APPROPRIATE CARE IN THE NICU

Hospitalization in the NICU constitutes a complex traumatic life event for the infant, which reflects the dual problem of exposure to traumatic events and the impact of those events on short- and long-term outcomes. The NCTSN published a very thorough review of complex trauma in children and adolescents (NCTSN Complex Trauma Task Force, 2003), which supports and substantiates the necessity of ensuring a trauma-informed age-appropriate approach to care in the NICU. Highlighting how trauma disrupts development through alterations in neurobiology sculpted by external experiences and in the absence of responsive caregiving, the affected individual develops altered reactivity to stress, which is usually severe and dysfunctional. Domains of impairment subsequent to early life experiences with complex trauma are listed in Table 3.1.

Maternal–infant interactions in the immediate postnatal period have a significant impact on neonatal outcomes. Consistency as well as quality of parental care benefits the infant's cognitive and social development (McEwen, 2011). Biologically programmed, the age-appropriate, expected experience for the neonate is the physical and emotional closeness of the parents. Even in the setting of prematurity and critical illness, there is a protective quality for brain development mediated by neural plasticity for infants whose parents are physically and emotionally available and present during the early postnatal period (Flacking et al., 2012).

Reynolds et al. (2013), in a prospective cohort study of high-risk infants less than 30 weeks gestational age, were able to demonstrate a statistically significant benefit of parental presence and holding in the NICU on neurobehavioral performance. Infants whose parents were present more often demonstrated better quality of movements and less excitability; infants who were held more by their parents, in addition to the aforementioned improvements, displayed less stress. Certainly confirming that parental

Table 3.1 *Domains of Impairment*

1. Attachment	5. Behavioral control
▪ Uncertainty about the reliability and predictability of the world ▪ Problems with boundaries ▪ Distrust and suspiciousness ▪ Social isolation ▪ Interpersonal difficulties ▪ Difficulty attuning to other people's emotional states ▪ Difficulty with perspective taking ▪ Difficulty enlisting other people as allies	▪ Poor modulation of impulses ▪ Self-destructive behavior ▪ Aggression against others ▪ Pathological self-soothing behaviors ▪ Sleep disturbances ▪ Eating disorders ▪ Substance abuse ▪ Excessive compliance ▪ Oppositional behavior ▪ Difficulty understanding and complying with rules ▪ Communication of traumatic past by reenactment in day-to-day behavior or play
2. Biology ▪ Sensorimotor developmental problems ▪ Hypersensitivity to physical contact ▪ Analgesia ▪ Problems with coordination, balance, body tone ▪ Difficulties localizing skin contact ▪ Somatization ▪ Increased medical problems across a wide span (e.g., pelvic pain, asthma, skin problems, autoimmune disorders, pseudoseizures) **3. Affect regulation** ▪ Difficulty with emotional self-regulation ▪ Difficulty describing feelings and internal experience ▪ Problems knowing and describing internal states ▪ Difficulty communicating wishes and desires	**6. Cognition** ▪ Difficulties in attention regulation and executive functioning ▪ Lack of sustained curiosity ▪ Problems with processing novel information ▪ Problems focusing on and completing tasks ▪ Problems with object constancy ▪ Difficulty planning and anticipating ▪ Problems understanding own contribution to what happens to them ▪ Learning difficulties ▪ Problems with language development ▪ Problems with orientation in time and space ▪ Acoustic and visual perceptual problems ▪ Impaired comprehension of complex visual-spatial patterns
4. Dissociation ▪ Distinct alterations in states of consciousness ▪ Amnesia ▪ Depersonalization and derealization ▪ Two or more distinct states of consciousness, with impaired memory for state-based events	**7. Self-concept** ▪ Lack of continuous, predictable sense of self ▪ Poor sense of separateness ▪ Disturbances of body image ▪ Low self-esteem ▪ Shame and guilt

Source: http://www.nctsn.org/sites/default/files/assets/pdfs/ComplexTrauma_All.pdf

presence is vital to infant well-being, the researchers uncovered that the majority of the parents (two-thirds) came to the NICU less than or equal to 5 days/week during the hospital stay. This important finding highlights the need for trauma-informed age-appropriate care in the NICU and operationalizing the attributes and criteria associated with the family-centered care core measure (Coughlin, 2011; Coughlin et al., 2009).

Smith et al. (2011) conducted a prospective cohort study of premature infants with a gestational age less than 30 weeks. Utilizing MRI, as well as neurobehavioral examinations at term equivalent, the researchers were able to demonstrate an association between exposure to stressors and brain structure and function. Specific findings included decreased frontal and parietal brain width, altered diffusion measures and functional connectivity in the temporal lobes, and abnormal motor behaviors found on neurobehavioral examination. The authors conclude that interventions to decrease or mitigate exposure to stressors in the NICU must be investigated.

Montirosso et al. (2012) completed a large multicenter, longitudinal study (Neonatal Adequate Care for Quality of Life [NEO-ACQUA]), which examined the quality of NICU developmental care and correlated that care to neurobehavioral performance in the study cohort. Inclusion criteria included infants with a gestational age less than or equal to 29 weeks and/or birth weight (BW) less than or equal to 1,500 g, no documented neurologic pathology, intraventricular hemorrhage (IVH) less than Grade III, no sensory deficits, and no malformation syndromes. Maternal demographics included mothers aged more than 18 years, with no history of psychiatric or cognitive pathology, no drug addiction, and not a single parent. Neurobehavioral performance was evaluated using the NICU Network Neurobehavioral Scale (NNS) administered when the study cohort reached clinical stability (postconceptual age range, 35 to 43 weeks). The Quality of Care Checklist (QCC) assessed a variety of procedures and practices related to developmental care. Following factor analysis of the QCC, two indices of developmental care were utilized: (a) infant-centered care practices (ICC)—parental presence, the frequency and duration of kangaroo care, and the presence of nursing interventions to support infant development by decreasing energy expenditure and promoting stability through containment, postural maneuvers, and a decrease in disturbing tactile stimulation; and (b) infant pain management (IPM)—frequency of pharmacologic and nonpharmacologic strategies for invasive medical procedures, the use of pharmacologic analgesia or sedation during continuous mechanical ventilation, the type of blood collection procedure employed, and the use of a clinical evaluation scale of newborn pain and/or written protocol for the management of newborn pain. After a very complete analysis of the data, the authors conclude that incorporating more developmental care practices and more pain control practices into a NICU's conventional care may promote neuromaturation of preterm infants, including an enhanced capacity for regulation and resilience.

TRAUMA-INFORMED AGE-APPROPRIATE CARE IN THE NICU

The term "trauma-informed age-appropriate care" is used to replace "developmental care" due to the latter's reputation and historical challenges in systematic adoption and implementation. Refining the clinical concept to reflect the latest research and evidence on developmental trauma provides the NICU clinician with a solid pan-scientific foundation that informs to transform the hospitalized infant's experience of care.

Incorporating the evidence-based best-practice strategies outlined in the National Association of Neonatal Nurses Guidelines for Age-Appropriate Care of the Premature and Critically Ill Hospitalized Infant in the NICU culture of care, the trauma associated with the NICU stay can be mitigated consistently and reliably. These guidelines, developed from the original work of Coughlin et al. (2009), will be outlined in detail in Section II.

CHAPTER 4: *Evidence-Based Care*

*T*he concept of evidence-based care (EBC) was introduced in the last decade of the 20th century. As more and more research and clinical data became available, medicine transitioned to a more systematic translation of research into clinical practice. Today, the multidisciplinary community of health care professionals serving patients around the globe embraces this concept. EBC is a practice strategy that incorporates the patient's values and expectations of the care delivery experience with clinician expertise grounded in the best available evidence (see Figure 4.1).

Despite the fact that evidence-based best practice has been around for two decades, challenges persist in the adoption and application of these best practices in the clinical setting. Ubbink, Guyatt, and Vermeulen (2013), using a systematic review design, summarized the self-reported appreciation and understanding of evidence-based best practice of nurses and physicians in 17 countries. Table 4.1 provides self-reported information regarding the attitudes of doctors and nurses toward evidence-based practice (EBP).

Table 4.2 lists barriers to the application of EBP in the clinical setting identified by these same doctors and nurses.

The authors conclude that the successful implementation of evidence-based best practices requires a multilevel approach spanning clinical practice, education, leadership, policy, and regulatory agencies.

THE JOINT COMMISSION AND EBP

To continuously improve health care for the public, in collaboration with other stakeholders, by evaluating healthcare organizations and inspiring them to excel in providing safe and effective care of the highest quality and value.—Joint Commission Mission Statement

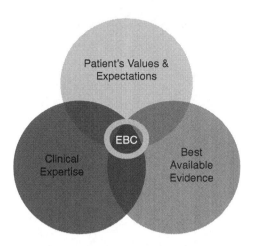

Figure 4.1 *Evidence-based care (EBC).*

The work of Dr. Ernest Codman during the first decade of the 20th century promoted hospital reform using patient care outcomes to inform practice improvement and practice change. This revolutionary approach to health care delivery established the framework for The Joint Commission (TJC), founded in 1951. TJC, a merger of the Hospital Standardization Program and the standards divisions of the American Hospital Association, the American Medical Association, and the Canadian Medical Association, is one of the preeminent organizations defining minimum standards of safety for hospital care across clinical, environmental, and competency domains.

TJC began to explore the development of performance measures related to specific disease entities in 1987 with its Agenda for Change, which came to be known as the ORYX initiative. This initiative was aimed at identifying performance metrics that would enable comparisons across and between health care organizations related to high-priority, disease-specific outcomes. At the turn of the 21st century, TJC, in collaboration with key stakeholders in health care including clinicians, hospital administrators, health care consumers, government and regulatory agencies, and medical associations, combined to identify focus areas for the development of core performance measures and associated evaluative criteria. The feedback from this diverse group of stakeholders provided the initial specifications for the core measure pilot-testing project that ensued.

Table 4.1 *Attitudes of Doctors and Nurses Toward EBP*

	Doctors' Median (Range)	Nurses' Median (Range)
Your current attitude toward EBP *Least positive (0) to extremely positive (100)*	72.3 (49–97)	66.7 (55–85)
Attitude of your colleagues toward EBP *Least positive (0) to extremely positive (100)*	61.0 (41–89)	48.0 (48–48)
How useful are research findings in daily practice? *Useless (0) to extremely useful (100)*	80.0 (46–97)	62.0 (34–82)
What percentage of your clinical practice is evidence based? *0% to 100%*	52.6 (40–80)	44.9 (44–46)
Practicing EBP improves patient care *Completely disagree (0) to fully agree (100)*	80.1 (52–97)	80.7 (74–87)
EBP is of limited value in clinical practice, because a scientific basis is lacking *Completely disagree (0) to fully agree (100)*	36.3 (3–43)	48.3 (48–49)
Implementing EBP, however worthwhile as an ideal, places another demand on already overloaded surgeons/nurses *Completely disagree (0) to fully agree (100)*	51.4 (37–56)	55.2 (17–61)
The amount of evidence is overwhelming *Completely disagree (0) to fully agree (100)*	53.5 (50–57)	No data
EBP fails in practice *Completely disagree (0) to fully agree (100)*	39.7 (15–84)	41.0 (39–63)
EBP is important for my profession *Completely disagree (0) to fully agree (100)*	68.3 (52–95)	61.6 (30–93)

Source: Ubbink et al. (2013).
EBP, evidence-based practice.

Table 4.2 *Barriers to Apply EBP as Mentioned by Doctors and Nurses*

Doctors and Nurses	
Lack of time to read evidence or implement new ideas	
Lack of facilities or resources	
Lack of staff experienced in EBP	
Lack of training in EBP	
EBP is insufficiently supported by staff and management	
Evidence is not easily available	
Unawareness of research	
Evidence is not generalizable to own setting	
Doctors	**Nurses**
Lack of evidence	Evidence is written in foreign language
Conflicting evidence	Lack of authority to change practice
Evidence is not incorporated in clinical practice	Statistics or research is unintelligible
EBP negatively impacts medical skills and freedom	Implications for practice are unclear

Source: Ubbink et al. (2013).
EBP, evidence-based practice.

Disease-Specific Core Measures

The core measure sets identified for the pilot work were selected based on their associated high mortality and included acute myocardial infarction (AMI), heart failure (HF), and community-acquired pneumonia (CAP). Evidence-based best practices in the medical and clinical management of these three disease entities were identified, standardized, and implemented in nine U.S. states (Connecticut, Michigan, Missouri, Rhode Island, Georgia, Texas, Virginia, California, and South Carolina).

Historically, disease management was highly variable and contingent on the individual practitioner's treatment style, knowledge base, past experience with various disease entities, and level of comfort with trying new strategies. The concept of disease prevention is relatively new, owing to epidemiologic shifts in leading causes of death from infectious origins to degenerative and man-made disease processes beginning in the mid-1900s (McLeroy & Crump, 1994). Hence, preventative medicine has taken a backseat to current medical practice strategies, which remain focused on symptom management of existing disease entities.

An example of the benefit of applying the core measure concept is represented in the management of cardiovascular disease, the leading cause of death across the globe and in the United States; current U.S. health care expenditure for cardiovascular disease alone exceeds $400 billion annually (Heidenreich et al., 2011). Implementing evidence-based best practices in the management of HF and AMI, described in the core measures, will dramatically reduce mortality associated with these two disease entities and significantly reduce the burden of disease associated with cardiovascular pathology.

Impact on Quality, Safety, and Practice

Adoption of evidence-based management strategies and a paradigm shift to prevention is imperative. In the setting of a burgeoning body of evidence that substantiates the efficacy of specific clinical practice strategies and therapeutic interventions with improved patient outcomes and reduced health care–associated costs, the adoption and standardization of evidence-based core measure practices become a key component of health care reform.

Jha, Orav, Li, and Epstein (2007) analyzed data from the Hospital Quality Alliance (HQA) program, which reported performance scores of over 4,000 U.S. hospitals related to compliance, with core measures for AMI, congestive HF, and CAP. Applying statistical analysis, the authors looked at associations between HQA performance and risk-adjusted mortality and concluded that hospitals with higher compliance with the performance metrics demonstrated a lower risk-adjusted mortality rate for their patient population. *EBC makes a difference.*

The relevance of this information highlights the clinical and economic benefits of adoption of evidence-based best practices in the delivery of safe, quality health care.

CORE MEASURES FOR AGE-APPROPRIATE CARE IN THE NICU

Unless someone like you cares a whole awful lot, nothing is going to get better.
It's not.—Dr. Seuss, *The Lorax*

The concept of core measures for age-appropriate care in the neonatal intensive care unit (NICU; originally core measures for developmental care) arose out of the need to standardize developmentally supportive care practices for neonatal clinicians worldwide. Developmental care practices have been inconsistently defined, adopted, and evaluated in clinical practice across the globe. Utilizing TJC concept of core measures and applying it to the disease-independent care needs of the premature and critically ill, hospitalized infants, Coughlin, Gibbins, and Hoath (2009) introduced minimum EBP expectations for neonatal intensive care clinicians. This new standard offers an objective reference point for the evaluation of evidence-based developmental care practices across various outcome metrics and also allows for cross-institutional comparison of developmental care programs.

The transition from the term developmental care to age-appropriate care links this practice care model to TJC's human resource standard requiring all staff to demonstrate competency in meeting the age-appropriate needs of the patient population served. This new terminology legitimizes and mandates the consistently reliable delivery of age-appropriate care to the premature and critically ill, hospitalized infant (Coughlin, 2011).

Disease-Independent Core Measures

Synthesizing and analyzing the available evidence for developmentally supportive care practices, Coughlin et al. (2009) categorized their findings into five core measure sets: (a) protected sleep, (b) pain and stress assessment and management, (c) developmental activities of daily living, (d) family-centered care, and (e) the healing environment. Each core measure set consists of three evidence-based attributes, and each attribute is comprised of corresponding evidence-based criteria.

Unlike TJC's core measures, focused on specific high-mortality/high-morbidity pathologic entities, the core measures for age-appropriate care focus on the human needs of the patient population served. These core needs underpin basic health and wellness for the hospitalized neonate across physiological, neurobiological, and psychoemotional domains. The core measures for age-appropriate care are the operational components of the conceptual model, the Universe of Developmental Care (UDC; Gibbins, Hoath, Coughlin, Gibbins, & Franck, 2008).

This conceptual model graphically portrays the centrality of the patient within the context of health care delivery. Theoretically and empirically grounded, the model emphasizes the concept of a shared care interface, where care is rendered and received. In the original representation, the infant is positioned at the center of the universe, encircled by an orbital plane that lists the physiological systems. It is a disturbance in one or more physiologic systems that brings the infant to the NICU. Proximal to this orbit, the sleep–wake cycle is positioned, representing the intimate relationship between physiologic integrity and sleep. Beyond this central core are nine care planets, displaying the various care activities that require patient interaction. The family is depicted as a comet, a dynamic ever-changing entity, positioned proximal to the infant encircled by the clinical staff and the health care organization.

In an updated and revised rendition of the UDC model, the Universe of Age-Appropriate Care extends its predecessor by including the infant's contribution to the care interaction by way of readiness cues and feedback, which share the sleep–wake orbit that envelops the integrity of the infant (Figure 4.2). In addition, the relationship of the health care team with the infant *and* family demonstrates the critical nature of a family-centered care approach and the need for partnership with parents and professionals to ensure the best possible outcomes for the infant–family dyad.

Through the consistently reliable delivery of evidence-based best practices in human caring, preventable, disease-independent morbidity can be reduced if not eliminated in this fragile patient population.

Based on estimates from 2005, the societal economic burden associated with prematurity in the United States is, at a minimum, $26.2 billion annually, encompassing medical costs, early intervention and special education expenses, as well as lost household and labor market productivity. This estimate does not capture costs associated with lifelong needs of the adult premature infant, including mental health services, adult hospitalizations, or ongoing medical services beyond childhood (National Research Council, 2007).

Minimizing the burden of disease associated with prematurity, which would also reduce some of the burden associated with mental illness associated with NICU survivors, requires the adoption of evidence-based best practices in the prevention and reduction of the deleterious effects of toxic stress and trauma on the developing critically ill neonate.

Core measures for age-appropriate care in the NICU quantify tangible caring nursing actions that have been previously "invisible" and link these actions with measurable outcomes. The nurse providing age-appropriate care interaction assesses the infant's readiness to engage in a caring exchange, based on sleep–wake state and infant feedback cues. In the example of an age-appropriate diaper change, the empathic nurse

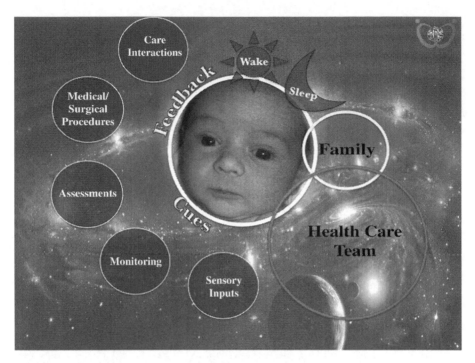

Figure 4.2 *Universe of age-appropriate care of the neonate.*

considers the light and sound levels within the immediate care area, constantly reading the infant's feedback cues, provides age-appropriate postural support during the procedure, assesses skin integrity, and engages the family to comfort and reassure the infant during this stress-laden yet seemingly simple task (Comaru & Miura, 2009; Monterosso, Kristjanson, Cole, & Evans, 2003; Newnham, Inder, & Milgrom, 2009).

Minimizing the stress and distress associated with the myriad of routine care interactions in the NICU by providing thoughtful, authentic age-appropriate caring, the quality and safety of the patient are ensured and morbidity associated with the NICU experience of care can be mitigated.

Impact on Quality, Safety, and Practice

The adoption of EBPs in the delivery of developmentally supportive care has yielded favorable outcomes beginning as early as the 1980s. The challenge has been in the variability in research methodology and measured outcome variables. Montirosso et al. (2012) examined the relationship between the neurobehavioral performance of very preterm infants and the level of NICU quality of developmental care. The researchers developed a Quality of Care Checklist (QCC) based on elements of the core measures for developmental care (Coughlin et al., 2009) and Als and Gilkerson's (1997) Neonatal Individualized Developmental Care and Assessment Program (NIDCAP)—specifically, the QCC assessed developmental care practices, policies toward parents, control of the environment, and infant pain management strategies. The study was a longitudinal, multicenter initiative in collaboration with 25 regional Level-III Italian NICUs. Inclusion criteria were gestational age less than or equal to 29 weeks and/or birth weight (BW) less than or equal to 1,500 g and no documented neurologic pathology. Neurobehavioral assessment was performed using the NICU Network Neurobehavioral Scale (NNNS) and infants were evaluated when they were clinically stable (postconceptual age ranged between 35 and 43 weeks). The results revealed that infants cared for in NICUs with high-quality, infant-centered care practices and high-quality infant pain management strategies exhibited higher attention and self-regulation skills, less excitability, and lower scores on hypotonicity and stress/abstinence than infants from low quality of care units. Also, for infants who received high-quality care related to infant pain management, these infants showed higher attention and arousal scores and lower scores on the lethargy and nonoptimal reflexes scales than preterm infants from low-care units (see Table 4.3 for definitions).

The authors conclude that the adoption and integration of evidence-based developmental care and pain management strategies into the

Table 4.3 *NNNS Terms and Definitions*

Attention	Ability to localize and track animate and inanimate auditory and visual stimuli
Self-regulation	Capacity to modulate arousal and organize motor activity
Excitability	High levels of motor, state, and physiologic reactivity
Hypotonicity	Hypotonic responses in arms, legs, trunk, or general tone
Stress/abstinence	Number of stress and abstinence signs observed during the exam
Arousal	Level of arousal maintained during the examination, including state and motor
Lethargy	Low levels of motor, state, and physiologic reactivity
Nonoptimal reflexes	Number of poor scores to elicited reflexes

NNNS, NICU Network Neurobehavioral Scale.

culture of care in the NICU promotes infant neuromaturation, including self-regulation and resilience.

SUMMARY

The provision of evidence-based best practices has a favorable impact on quality and patient safety for both disease-dependent and disease-independent processes. Challenges in the translation of research into clinical practice must be investigated and resolved.

Principles of EBP for Patient Safety

- First, consider the context and engage health care personnel who are at the point of care in selecting and prioritizing patient safety initiatives.
- Second, illustrate through qualitative or quantitative data (e.g., near misses, sentinel events, adverse events, injuries from adverse events) the reason the organization and individuals within the organization should commit to an evidence-based safety practice topic.
- Third, didactic education alone is never enough to change practice; one-time education on a specific safety initiative is not enough.
- Fourth, the context of EBP improvements in patient safety needs to be addressed at each step of the implementation process; piloting the change in practice is essential to determine the fit between the EBP patient safety information/innovation and the setting of care delivery.
- Finally, it is important to evaluate the processes and outcomes of implementation. Users and stakeholders need to know that the efforts to improve patient safety have a positive impact on quality of care. (Martha G. Titler, 2008)

Chapter 11 in Section III will present patient quality and safety outcomes associated with the implementation of the core measures for age-appropriate care in the NICU.

CHAPTER 5: *The Importance of Nursing's Legacy of Caring in the NICU*

LEGACY OF CARING IN NURSING

The concept of caring has been an essential element of nursing practice since the profession's founder, Florence Nightingale (1860), described the tenets of professional nursing practice in her *Notes on Nursing—What It Is and What It Is Not* (Table 5.1).

Professional nursing practice has grown, matured, and evolved over the past 150 years since Nightingale's first band of nurses cared for the wounded and infirmed soldiers of the Crimean War in Scutari, Turkey, in 1855. Advanced practice nurse practitioners, clinical specialists, nurse scientists, and nurse researchers represent the diversity and growth of professional nursing practice, but regardless of which path is taken, nurses share a philosophical and scientific common denominator—caring for other. In our own unique way we become the "Lady With the Lamp" as we watch over and minister to those vulnerable individuals we serve day and night, bearing witness to their experience and easing their distress and discomfort through presence, intention, and the art and science of nursing (Naef, 2006; Schoenhofer, 2002).

The whole is greater than the sum of its parts.—Aristotle

What does this quotation from Aristotle mean for professional nursing practice? In the setting of innumerable tasks and competing priorities, nurses tend to economize on their communications and references to patients. For example, instead of referring to the infant born at 25 weeks

Table 5.1 *Nightingale's Tenets and Modern Correlates*

Nightingale's Tenets	Modern Nursing Concept Correlates
Ventilation and warming Light Cleanliness of rooms and walls Health of houses Noise Bed and bedding Personal cleanliness	Physical environment
Variety Chattering of hopes and advices	Psychological environment
Taking food What food?	Nutritional status
Petty management Observation of the sick	Nursing care planning and management

gestation with respiratory distress syndrome and patent ductus arteriosus, we may simply refer to this individual as "the 25 weeker," or the individual born at 36 weeks gestation hospitalized for a diaphragmatic hernia may be regarded as "the diaphragm." A similar phenomenon is seen in adult clinical settings where the patient may be referred to as "the gallbladder in room 4" or "the hernia in room 7." Although these references may save some time in our communications and explanations, reducing the individual to his or her diagnostic condition demeans and diminishes their humanity.

Over time, this "efficiency" erodes our relationship with the patient, which undermines our professional integrity and identity (Nolan, 2013). The hospitalized individual has needs that extend well beyond his or her primary diagnosis and include the need to be recognized and respected as a person; the need to be cared for in a healing space that promotes rest and recovery; the need for social support from family or other personally significant relationships; and the need for experienced pain and stress to be managed effectively, consistently, and reliably—the hospitalized individual needs to feel "cared for" (Carter, 2009; Eggenberger & Nelms, 2007; Jarrín, 2012).

Nursing science is not about disease management per se, but instead is about managing the human experience of disease. There are many medical conditions that require hospitalization but may not necessarily be cured, but the one thing that we, as professional nurses, can bring to the patient's experience is ourselves, our presence, the noble responsibility of bearing witness to the suffering of another and alleviating distress through compassion and authentic being (Favero, Pagliuca, & Lacerda, 2013; Naef, 2006; Watson, 2003). It is through the therapeutic use of self that the nurse makes a difference, and *becomes* the difference for the patient.

The art and science of nursing do not conform to reductionism; nursing is founded on the acknowledgment that the person *is* "greater than the sum of their parts." "Nurses are morally obligated to protect their patients from the vulnerability associated with illness" (Hogan, 2013) as well as vulnerabilities associated with the experience of care in managing the illness. *First do no harm.*

Neonatal nursing, beginning at the turn of the 20th century, has seen dramatic changes in the medical and surgical management of premature and critically ill newborns. The introduction of literally lifesaving treatments and revolutionary medical technologies has dramatically reduced mortality in this fragile patient population. Given this 100-year history, it has been a mere 40 years since the idea of responding to the developmental human needs of this special population was introduced to neonatology by Dr. Heidelise Als and her colleagues. Today, neonatal intensive care units (NICUs) continue to struggle to consistently and reliably merge the developmental human requisites of the hospitalized neonate with diagnosis-driven needs.

Responding to this perceived dichotomy is the role of the professional neonatal nurse. Caring for the human needs of an individual is not mutually exclusive to managing his or her medical/surgical needs. This is the legacy of caring in nursing.

> *Apprehension, uncertainty, waiting, expectation, fear of surprise, do a patient more harm than any exertion.*—Florence Nightingale

NURSING THEORY

Theory of nursing science defines, describes, and explains phenomena specific to nursing practice. The profession has been honored by a multitude of nurse theorists, researchers, and scientists who have made substantial contributions to the body of nursing knowledge defining and elaborating on the roles, responsibilities, and scope of nursing practice. Common themes identified in nursing theory include the person or patient, the environment (internal and external), health and wellness, and the role of the nurse. These themes arise from a locus of caring, comfort, and restoration. Nightingale introduces this in her original nursing framework and it has been woven into the theoretical frameworks of her successors over the past 150 years.

Jean Watson introduced her theory of transpersonal caring or human caring science in 1979 and has pioneered the research investigating and describing the impact of caring on the patient's experience as well as the nurse's professional satisfaction. Both Nightingale and Watson identify caring as a quintessential component of professional nursing practice and have linked caring actions, attitudes, and behaviors with measurable outcomes across physical, psychosocial, and spiritual domains.

Florence Nightingale

The nurse is responsible for creating and maintaining an environment
conducive to the healing process.—Florence Nightingale

Florence Nightingale, the founder of professional nursing, established the first theoretical framework that guided early nursing professionals in ministering to the sick and infirmed. Her tenets of professional nursing remain relevant for today's practicing nurses and include a focus on the physical and psychological environment, the role of nutrition in recovery and wellness, and the nurse's role in assessing, critically thinking, planning, and managing the patient's experience of disease to restore health and wellness.

Nightingale's tenets for nursing practice respond to the human experience of disease at a fundamental level. Within the context of the available medical resources of her time, these caring actions highlight the quintessential role nursing plays in facilitating recovery from illness and the restoration of wellness through authentic caring for body, mind, and spirit.

Recognized as a clinical audit pioneer, Nightingale set the standard for professional nursing practice to continuously evaluate and document the efficacy of various nursing and medical interventions on the patient's biopsychosocial well-being. This not only enabled the professional nurse to individualize care based on the patient's responses and progress, but also provided the substrate to evaluate patient outcomes retrospectively through medical record audit. Nightingale was able to assemble quantitative data related to nursing practices from patients' records to lobby for care improvements in the British Health System (Selanders, 2005). Today's nurse is compelled to continue this critical task if nursing is to survive.

Continuously validating the quality of experience and lifesaving benefits of authentic nurse caring (genuine nursing) in the nurse–patient relationship plays a key role in health care reform.

> If we are caught in the devil's bargain whereby we spend increasing amounts on technology but in order to protect against major cost overruns simultaneously cut budgets for frontline staff then we may be in jeopardy of undermining the "care" in our healthcare services. Should we uncritically travel down this wide and well-lit avenue rather than preserving a critical skepticism to protect the efficacious and humane treatment of our population's health, we run the risk of merely emulating a giant and highly profitable industrial conveyor belt rather than a humane institution consistent with the Hippocratic oath. (Coughlan, 2006)

Nightingale's model for nursing practice reflects her philosophical approach to the nurse–patient relationship as a continuous and dynamic exchange of information and thoughtful interventions framed by an authentic holistic caring for other (Figure 5.1).

Nightingale's approach to the nurse–patient encounter resonates with the world of neonatal nursing. With an emphasis on the patient (person), nursing actions are aimed at environmental modifications that benefit the patient, not the technology. Person-centered care (or, more accurately, family-centered care) is reflected in the core measures for age-appropriate care based on the Nightingale legacy.

Jean Watson

Caring is the essence of nursing.—Jean Watson

To validate the concept of caring as a critical element in nursing, Dr. Jean Watson embarked on a groundbreaking approach to nursing—one that legitimized the art and science of caring in nursing. The science of caring links human emotional experiences with scientific knowledge and methodologies that demonstrate the crucial role caring plays in healing.

Watson boldly professes that the role of health care professionals extends beyond a "detached scientific endeavor" but is "a life-giving and life-receiving endeavor for humanity" (Watson, 2005). Coining the term "transpersonal," Watson illustrates the therapeutic use of self in care interactions with patients and colleagues. Watson outlined 10 fundamental elements that define the nurse–patient relationship; these "caritas processes" define and guide caring interactions for the professional nurse (Table 5.2).

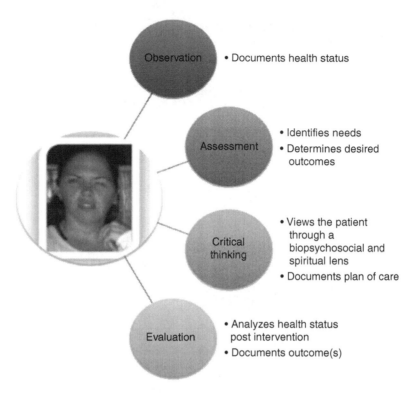

Figure 5.1 *Adaptation of Nightingale's model of nursing practice.*

Table 5.2 *Watson's 10 Caritas Processes*

1. Embrace altruistic values and practice loving kindness with self and others.
2. Instill faith and hope and honor others.
3. Be sensitive to self and others by nurturing individual beliefs and practices.
4. Develop helping–trusting–caring relationships.
5. Promote and accept positive and negative feelings as you authentically listen to another's story.
6. Use creative scientific problem-solving methods for caring decision making.
7. Share teaching and learning that addresses individual needs and comprehension styles.
8. Create a healing environment for the physical and spiritual self, which respects human dignity.
9. Assist with basic physical, emotional, and spiritual human needs.
10. Open to mystery and allow miracles to enter.

These caritas processes describe the transpersonal caring moment grounded by the philosophical and ethical work of Levinas and Logstrup, who frame Watson's treatise on human caring science. This perspective links the work of nursing with universal concepts acknowledging our shared humanity and juxtaposes the work of nursing with metaphysics.

This juxtaposition of nursing and metaphysics highlights the complexity and pervasiveness of our connection with other and how the caring moment is more than what meets the eye. "Everything that exists is inseparable...Remembering that we are energy beings designed to perceive and translate energy into neural code may help [us] become more aware of [our] energy dynamic and intuition" (Curtin, 2010).

Watson's concept of transpersonal caring highlights our inseparability with other and the intimate reciprocity of the caring interaction.

Transpersonal refers to an intersubjectivity of the human to human relationship in which the person of the nurse influences and is influenced by another person. Both are fully present in the moment and feel a bond with one another. They share a phenomenological field that becomes part of the life history, and both are co-participants in becoming the now and the future. (Watson, 2012)

This transpersonal model has been introduced to neonatal nursing through the recent conceptual model, The Universe of Developmental Care, which attempts to graphically represent a patient-centered experience for the hospitalized infant and highlights a shared interface of care. It is at this interface, likened to a Mobius strip (Figure 5.2), that care is rendered and received: "The surface is not a barrier separating self and nonself or brain and environment, but a seamless union of both" (Gibbins, Hoath, Coughlin, Gibbins, & Franck, 2008).

Watson entreats the professional nurse to acknowledge this union with other, recognizing the inherent vulnerability of the individuals served in the caring moment and engage in activities that cultivate and sustain caring for self and other—as is our calling.

(Watson) acknowledge(s) the work of Knud Logstrup, a Danish philosopher who mirrors views similar to Levinas, but from the metaphor of "Hand," in that he reminds us that:

"Holding another person's life in one's hand, endows this metaphor with a certain emotional power...that we have the power to determine the direction of something in another person's

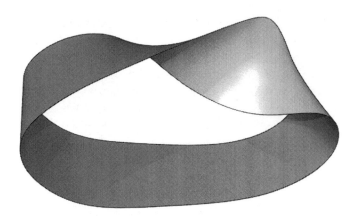

Figure **5.2** *Mobius strip. A surface with only one side and one boundary is a metaphor for the simple yet complex nature of the patient–nurse interaction at the shared interface of care.*

life...we're to a large extent inescapably dependent upon one another...we are mutually and in a most immediate sense in one another's power." (Watson, 2003)

It is difficult to refute the vulnerability of the premature and critically ill infant and, for many of these individuals, they literally can be held within the hand of the neonatal nurse. The magnitude of this reality must exemplify the magnificent power of caring, and, as Watson extends, love for other.

EVALUATING CARING

> *Caring is a complex of attitudes and behaviours that reflects and conveys the health care provider's respect for the patient as an autonomous person, with values, goals, feelings, and beliefs that cannot be inferred simply from a medical diagnosis or record, yet which have a legitimate bearing on what ought to be done for that patient in the context of treatment. Caring is thus a fundamentally communicative phenomenon, absorbing significant time and effort. It requires the [realization] that what the patient thinks, wants and fears is important, and can only be discovered through visible effort.* — Samuel Gorovitz

Caring is a dynamic and multifaceted concept. As such, clinicians struggle in measuring the impact of authentic caring experiences in the clinical setting. In the NICU, oftentimes clinicians perceive age-appropriate care as a nicety and something to implement once the infant is stable; this inconsistency makes outcome data difficult to interpret and does not exemplify the tenets of professional nursing as outlined by Nightingale and Watson. It is when the infant is at his or her most vulnerable and most frightened that authentic caring through the adoption and consistently reliable provision of age-appropriate care practices allays the infant's fear, and he or she is comforted and supported through the acute and convalescent phases of his or her hospitalization.

In order to care authentically for these tiny, fragile individuals, it becomes incumbent on the neonatal clinician to demonstrate competence and confidence in reading the infant's biobehavioral cues of communication, as these individuals are hospitalized during their preverbal stage of development. This being stated, communication is not solely achieved through observation and feedback, as there are medical conditions and pharmacological interventions that may blunt or obliterate the infant's capacity to exhibit communicative cues. It is at this juncture that the professional nurse must draw upon his or her empathy and intersubjective awareness of other to determine the appropriate "next action"; it is not sufficient to assume, in the absence of infant cues, that a care interaction should be initiated or to proceed.

Evaluating caring interactions is similar to evaluating the efficacy of any interaction (or intervention). Through the therapeutic use of self, the nurse can assess the infant's level of comfort, distress, anxiety, and fear, responding thoughtfully and consistently. This assessment can be made using the biobehavioral cues of the infant *or* through the empathic relationship with other, applying Watson's transpersonal caring framework. The neonatal nurse, guided by nursing process and nursing ethics, manages the unfolding experience of the hospitalized infant and provides evidence-based age-appropriate caring strategies to create an environment conducive to optimal physiological, neurobiological, and psychoemotional recovery.

Caring Metrics for the NICU

Although there is a fairly solid and still growing body of research documenting the benefits of developmentally supportive care practices (age-appropriate care) in the NICU, the consistently reliable adoption and true standardization of this practice strategy have remained elusive. Concept analysis of developmental care as well as evidence-based components of developmental care has been presented in the nursing literature demonstrating the necessity of this practice strategy; however, in the absence of a systematic approach to cultural transformation with clearly articulated performance expectations, inconsistency in managing the age-appropriate needs of this vulnerable population will persist (Aita & Snider, 2003; Byers, 2003).

According to Aucott, Donohue, Atkins, and Allen (2002), neurodevelopmental care interventions encompass the NICU design and environment (light and sound), supportive positioning and handling practices, the provision of nonnutritive sucking, family participation, breast-feeding, kangaroo care, and pain management. Delineating a comprehensive list of caregiving categories and interventions is insufficient to change practice. This type of approach to developmentally supportive care is analogous to giving someone directions by simply telling him the destination. Of course, in today's world one only needs the destination and a smartphone to figure out the route, but even then the smartphone often provides several options to reach the destination. If I choose Option 1, and my colleague chooses Option 2, and the night nurse chooses Option 3, collectively we are not creating a consistent experience of care for the infant; we are not creating a trusting milieu.

Montirosso et al. (2012) struggled with clarity of a consistent definition for developmental care, prompting the creation of the Neonatal Adequate Care for Quality of Life (NEO-ACQUA) study group, which developed a quality of care checklist based on the work of Coughlin, Gibbins, and Hoath (2009; Figure 5.3) and Dr. Heidelise Als's Neonatal Individualized Developmental Care and Assessment Program (NIDCAP). This checklist served as a clear, objective, and evidence-based guide to assess the quality of developmental care provided across their 25-NICU network. As presented in the previous chapter, very preterm infants'

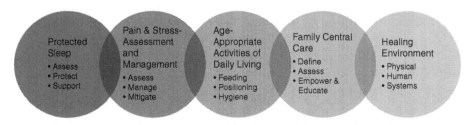

Figure 5.3 *Attributes of the core measures for age-appropriate care.*

neurobehavioral stability was statistically significantly enhanced in NICUs that delivered a higher quality of developmental care. The success in this study was the clarity in criteria and the culture of care.

The core measures for age-appropriate care delineate five domains of recurring themes found in the literature regarding developmentally supportive care and quality caring practices in neonatal populations. These five domains include (a) the healing environment, (b) protected sleep, (c) assessment and management of pain and stress, (d) activities of daily living (positioning, feeding, skin care/hygiene), and (e) family-centered care (Coughlin et al., 2009). Within each domain are clearly articulated, evidence-based attributes and associated criteria regarding the practice expectation, which will be described in Section II.

Why Is There Such Difficulty in Standardizing This Clearly Beneficial, Evidence-Based Practice Model in the NICU?

Hendricks-Muñoz and Prendergast (2007), using a 12-point questionnaire, investigated neonatal nurse–perceived barriers to implementing developmental care across 24 regional hospitals in the greater New York City area. With a return rate of 86%, 93% of respondents indicated developmental care was essential to the care of their fragile patient population, yet 86% believed their NICU was not providing optimal developmental care. The most frequently cited barriers were related to the human environment: physician leadership, nursing leadership, and nurse colleagues.

Mosqueda et al. (2013), using a questionnaire design, sought to understand the necessary requirements and obstacles to implementing Als's NIDCAP. The study results also affirmed challenges at the level of the human environment, including coordination among the multidisciplinary team serving the NICU.

In the absence of clarity of performance expectations, clinicians will provide care that they believe is best for the individuals served. This belief is based on their existing knowledge level as well as past experiences and observations. This model of care delivery, although well intended, creates a milieu of mistrust and confusion at the patient interface. The core measures for developmentally supportive care, now referred to as core measures for age-appropriate care (Coughlin, 2011), were developed to create consistency in performance expectations. "Clearly defined, measurable evidence-based clinical practice criteria (as outlined by the core measures) provide an objective reference point for developmental care practice improvement in the NICU" (Coughlin et al., 2009).

Next Steps for Caring in the NICU

In the tradition of Nightingale and Watson, it is our nursing legacy, and indeed a nursing imperative, to provide responsive, authentic caring to the individuals we serve, beyond their diagnostic conditions. Caring actions, attitudes, and behaviors must become hardwired into the culture of care in the NICU.

Embracing a systematic and transdisciplinary approach to transform the experience of care of the premature and critically ill, hospitalized infant is not easy but is clearly the right thing to do. This concept of "the right thing to do" finds its roots in social justice and advocacy, seen through the lens of professional nursing (Buettner-Schmidt & Lobo, 2012; Paquin, 2011). Advocating for the consistently reliable provision of age-appropriate care in the NICU is a moral imperative that impacts global public health.

Nightingale laid the foundation for the role of nursing to uphold social justice, and that as a profession dedicated to serving other, it was paramount that those who enter the profession truly understand their role and responsibilities.

> Nightingale (1915 edition) was acutely aware that if nurses were to successfully fulfill their role as "guardians of the community's interests," they needed to: guard themselves against becoming "stagnant women" (p. 5), engage in constant self-directed learning and work to improve their "own mind and character every day" (p. 50), develop proficiency and always [strive] to "know the reason why" (p. 70), and resist becoming enamored with "the good opinion which men have of you" else fall prey "to neglecting themselves" and become conceited and arrogant (p. 58). (Johnstone, 2011)

In reviewing the literature to gain insight into the barriers to adopt and systematically integrate evidence-based, age-appropriate care strategies into the culture of care in the NICU, the human environment is a recurring challenge. Individual clinician explanations for this challenge/resistance to adopt age-appropriate care practices span a range of rationalizations that on the surface seem plausible, but when questioned in the light of new and emerging evidence fail to be substantive.

Changing a culture of care where the patient and family are truly the central focus for care is a dramatic paradigm shift in today's corporate health care structure; it is difficult to stay focused on the primacy of nursing, but, when all is said and done, it is our legacy and our raison d'être.

> Ethics is an integral part of the foundation of nursing. Nursing has a distinguished history of concern for the welfare of the sick, injured, and vulnerable and for social justice. This concern is embodied in the provision of nursing care to individuals and the community. Nursing encompasses the prevention of illness, the alleviation of suffering, and the protection, promotion, and restoration of health in the care of individuals, families, groups, and communities. Nurses act to change those aspects of social structures that detract from health and well-being. Individuals who become nurses are expected not only to adhere to the ideals and moral norms of the profession but also to embrace them as a part of what it means to be a nurse. The ethical tradition of nursing is self-reflective, enduring, and distinctive. A code of ethics makes explicit the primary goals, values, and obligations of the profession. (Preface to the 2010 ANA Code of Ethics; American Nurses Association, 2010)

Nursing must champion this paradigm shift and restore and ensure the provision of age-appropriate quality caring experiences for premature and critically ill, hospitalized infants.

SECTION II: *Core Measures for Trauma-Informed Age-Appropriate Care*

CHAPTER 6: *The Healing Environment*

WHAT IS A HEALING ENVIRONMENT?

The concept of a healing environment has reemerged in modern health care as a major contributor to recovery, patient satisfaction, and patient safety (Seifert & Hickman, 2005). Hospitals historically were designed for efficiency in the provision of high-tech, state-of-the-art medical care and consequently have become noisy, hectic, stressful environments that compromise healing and safety (Schweitzer, Gilpin, & Frampton, 2004).

Nightingale defined the elements of a healing environment in her *Notes on Hospitals, Notes on Nursing,* and other formal communications to her nurses. These elements ring true today. They include the physical space (bedding, cleanliness and tidiness, light, noise, ventilation, privacy, and aesthetics) as well as the human environment (caring, presence, communication, collaboration, respect, and trust). Selanders (2010) restates Nightingale's canons of nursing practice: "The nurse is responsible for maintaining the environment in such a manner as to maintain the health of the patient."

As defined by the core measures for age-appropriate care and framed by Nightingale's model for nursing practice, the healing environment is comprised of the physical, human, and system attributes (Coughlin, 2011; Coughlin et al., 2009). In this chapter, you will be introduced to a revision of this core measure where the physical environment encompasses the sensory milieu, the physical space, and the aesthetics; the human environment is comprised of communication, collaboration, and caring; and the systems environment includes

Table 6.1 *Healing Environment Attributes and Criteria*

A soothing, spacious, and aesthetically pleasing environment conducive to rest, healing, and recovery	1. Sensory milieu ensures light and sound levels are maintained within recommended ranges as well as positive age-appropriate tactile, vestibular, olfactory, gustatory, auditory, and visual experiences 2. The space provides for privacy, parenting, and interpersonal experiences, and the provision of safe, quality patient care 3. Art, aesthetics, and space convey a healing environment and respect for human dignity
A collaborative health care team that emanates teamwork, mindfulness, and caring	1. Collaboration—Interprofessional rounds occur weekly and ensure consistency in care across all disciplines 2. Caring—Direct care providers demonstrate caring behaviors that include adherence to hand hygiene protocols, cultural sensitivity, open listening skills, and a sensitive relationship orientation 3. Communication—Verbal, written, and behavioral (nonverbal) communication is respectful, complete, and patient centered
Evidence-based policies, procedures, and resources are available to sustain the healing environment over time	1. Standards—Core measures for age-appropriate care provide the standard of care for all patient care encounters 2. Resources—Both human and material resources to support the implementation of age-appropriate care are in place 3. Accountability—All staff hold themselves and their colleagues accountable for the provision of evidence-based, age-appropriate care

best-practice standards, accountability, and both human and material resources.

Table 6.1 outlines the attributes and criteria for this very important core measure.

Why Is the Healing Environment Important in the NICU?

The importance of the healing environment in neonatal intensive care is revealed in the research, demonstrating how early adverse experiences impact brain development. These adverse experiences emanate from the environment of care and the caregiving encounter. As described in Chapter 2, the premature and critically ill infant is profoundly vulnerable and susceptible across physiological, neurobiological, and psychological domains. The physical, human, and systems components of the environment frame the infant–family dyad's hospital experience and set expectations that guide the provision of evidence-based best practice in quality human caring.

Consequences of an Unhealthy Environment of Care

Consequences associated with an unhealthy environment of care include breaches in quality as well as patient safety in both the short and long term for the patient, family, clinician, and organization. Specific patient consequences include sleep deprivation from excessive noise and light, development of tactile vulnerability and sensory integration challenges, as well as hearing impairments (Kamdar, Needham, & Collop, 2012; Nakos, 2012; Wachman & Lahav, 2011; Weiss & Wilson, 2006).

Burnout, poor communication, lack of teamwork, and compromised patient safety are additional consequences associated with an unhealthy human environment of care impacting the patient, the professional, and the organization (Leape et al., 2012; Ohlinger, Brown, Laudert, Swanson, & Fofah, 2003; Spence Laschinger, Leiter, Day, & Gilin, 2009). With regard to the systems environment, "the art of inconsistency" and a paucity of accountability compromise the environment of care, patient safety goals, and staff satisfaction (Golec, 2009).

EVIDENCE-BASED CARE STRATEGIES TO SUPPORT A HEALING ENVIRONMENT

The Physical Environment

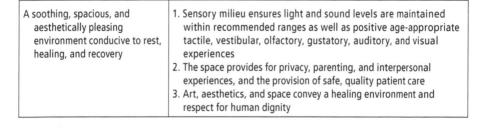

A soothing, spacious, and aesthetically pleasing environment conducive to rest, healing, and recovery	1. Sensory milieu ensures light and sound levels are maintained within recommended ranges as well as positive age-appropriate tactile, vestibular, olfactory, gustatory, auditory, and visual experiences 2. The space provides for privacy, parenting, and interpersonal experiences, and the provision of safe, quality patient care 3. Art, aesthetics, and space convey a healing environment and respect for human dignity

From touch to movement, noise to light, taste to smell, neonatal intensive care unit (NICU) nurses are poised to moderate and manage the noxious components of sensory stimulation to which premature and critically ill infants are exposed, and create nurturing, age-appropriate sensory experiences.

Each sensory system has its own developmental sequence linked to underlying neural architecture. Sensory systems develop in close

Table 6.2 *Sensory System Development*

System	Maturation
Tactile	Sensory nerve fibers functional by 11 weeks
Vestibular	Functional by 21 weeks
Gustatory	Taste buds emerge by 20 weeks
Olfactory	Nasal structure and associated components in place by 8 weeks
Auditory	Structurally and functionally complete by 24 weeks
Visual	Structurally complete by 40 weeks, function evolves over the next several months postnatal

association with each other to facilitate coordination and functional integration that are required for optimal development (Graven & Browne, 2008a; Table 6.2). Tactile sensory nerve fibers are functional by 11 weeks gestation, and there is a higher density of these nerve fibers located in the perioral and perianal areas as well as the palms of the hands and soles of the feet. Having knowledge of this embryological reality informs the NICU clinician to understand the heightened vulnerability of these regions to procedural touch and manage these experiences compassionately and consistently.

Following birth and NICU admission of the critically ill infant (regardless of gestational age), there is a significant amount of procedurally driven tactile stimulation linked to the infant's severity of illness and need for intensive care. The stress, fear, and vulnerability associated with repeated procedural and caregiving touch can be managed effectively with several nonpharmacological strategies, including kangaroo care, nonnutritive sucking, containment, gentle touch, reassuring vocalizations, and massage, to name a few (Bahman Bijari, Iranmanesh, Eshghi, & Baneshi, 2012; Field, Diego, & Hernandez-Reif, 2010; Jefferies, 2012; Pillai Riddell et al., 2011; Seltzer, Ziegler, & Pollak, 2010).

The critically ill infant often requires excessive manipulation and invasion of the oral pharyngeal cavity. Endotracheal intubation and insertion of a feeding tube (either orally or nasally) are profoundly noxious events. Stabilizing and affixing these tubes create an additional negative sensory experience that, when combined, have long-term effects on successful oral feeding. It is not uncommon for NICU graduates to develop oral aversion once they become volitional eaters; these individuals develop failure to thrive and require gastrostomy tube placement and protracted therapy to reestablish minimal success in oral feeding (Quinn, 2008). Evidence-based caring interventions to manage these multisensory procedures include premedication for endotracheal intubation with a facilitated tuck; the use of nonpharmacological strategies to manage the stress and distress associated with feeding tube placement; the judicious use of tape or other stabilizing devices to secure these tubes; and the mindful use of nonpharmacological strategies when removing the tape, the stabilizing device, and/or the tubes (Carbajal, Eble, & Anand, 2007; Kumar, Denson, & Mancuso, 2010; McCullough, Halton, Mowbray, & Macfarlane, 2008; Nanavati, Balan, & Kabra, 2013; Nimbalkar, Sinojia, & Dongara, 2013; Pandey, Datta, & Rehan, 2013; Pillai Riddell et al., 2011).

In addition to managing noxious sensory experiences, the age-appropriate neonatal nurse can also provide procedure-independent, positive sensory experiences. One such experience is the use of breast milk for oral care. Thibeau and Boudreaux (2013), in a retrospective descriptive study, explored the benefits of breast milk for oral care in mechanically ventilated, very low birth weight (VLBW) premature infants. Their findings suggest that the use of breast milk for oral care is feasible and safe as part of a ventilator-associated pneumonia (VAP) prevention bundle.

Taste buds emerge at 20 weeks gestation and the fetus sucks and swallows an average of 1 L of amniotic fluid daily. The molecular components of amniotic fluid from a flavor and odor makeup are similar to maternal breast milk and maternal perspiration and represent early sensory learning for postnatal adaptation (Ventura & Worobey, 2013).

Exposing the critically ill infant to familiar gustatory and olfactory stimulants such as breast milk and maternal scent provides familiar sensory experiences that can allay infant stress and anxiety and facilitate attachment and bonding (Flacking et al., 2012).

Clinical observations of externally applied vestibular stimulation in the absence of proprioceptive support result in significant autonomic instability in many critically ill infants (Limperopoulos et al., 2008). Position changes and location transfers (bed to scale, bed to transport incubator, bed to parents) can be disruptive and a source of biological stress. NICU clinicians must exercise presence and patience to minimize the associated distress of these activities to the patient. Movements should be slow, deliberate, and supported. When transferring the infant, the infant should be brought close into the chest of the clinician to provide proprioceptive input and a reference point for the movement. When transferring an infant from the incubator or warming table to a parent, ensure that all the lines, tubes, wires, and so forth are aligned within the infant's nest in preparation for the transfer. The infant should not be transferred without some form of swaddling support or nest to maintain postural alignment, safety, and security for the infant (Ludington-Hoe, Morgan, & Abouelfettoh, 2008)

A discussion of evidence-based practices (EBPs) regarding the NICU sensory milieu would not be complete without a review of the auditory and visual aspects of the physical environment and recommendations for improvement.

The World Health Organization (WHO) recommends that average background noise in hospitals should not exceed 30 dB; this is equivalent to a soft whisper. Needless to say, the noise levels in hospitals, and especially in NICUs, are much greater than this. The U.S. Environmental Protection Agency (EPA) in 1974 issued recommendations that daytime hospital noise levels not exceed 45 dB and nighttime levels not exceed 35 dB. The American Academy of Pediatrics (AAP) recommends NICU noise levels to be less than 45 dB and NICU light levels less than 646 lux (60 foot-candles).

Excessive noise not only affects physiologic integrity of *all* the individuals within the environment but also compromises communication and poses a safety hazard (Choiniere, 2010). The AAP Committee on Environmental Health (1997) issued a comprehensive review of the hazards of noise on the fetus and newborn, including noise-induced hearing loss and hypoxemia. Recommendations to manage the sound levels have included reducing noise levels associated with manufactured equipment, routinely monitoring sound levels both in and around incubators, and employing simple strategies to reduce noise exposure to the infant, such as not placing equipment on or in the incubator, avoiding tapping or writing on the tops of the incubators, and closing incubator portholes gently. Additional strategies to reduce noise are moving nonclinical conversations away from the patient care area and speaking in soft voices when in the care area, promptly responding to alarms, eliminating intercoms and overhead paging systems, and employing a vibrate-only pagers and cell phones policy.

Strategies regarding the light environment can be challenging based on the diversity in lighting needs across patients and staff. Although recommendations for individuals less than 30 weeks are for decreased light exposure, critically ill term infants benefit from a cycled lighting strategy, and then there are the lighting needs of clinicians to deliver safe patient care. Meeting these needs requires creativity, engagement, and empowerment of bedside clinicians.

All neonates should be protected from direct light to the eyes. Individuals with a gestational age less than 30 weeks should always be protected from bright light due to the immaturity of the pupillary reflex, which is unable to reflexively constrict in response to light (Osorio, Hertle, Painter, & Hinch, 2009; Robinson & Fielder, 1990). Between 30 and 35 weeks there is variability in the responsiveness of the premature pupil to light. Individuals undergoing eye examination with chemical dilation, in addition to procedural pain management, should have protective eye wear in place postexamination, with length of wear time determined by the medication's half-life (Mitchell, Green, Jeffs, & Roberson, 2011; Samra & McGrath, 2009).

Additional hazards related to the NICU environment include exposure to electromagnetic fields, radiation, plasticizers, and inactive ingredients in medications (Lai & Bearer, 2008; Whittaker et al., 2009). The provision of age-appropriate care in the NICU must mitigate and manage the deleterious effects of the entire NICU environment. Success in creating a safe, nurturing milieu that is responsive to the developmental, physiological, psychoemotional, and environmental needs of this fragile population requires commitment from collaborative clinicians—the human environment of care.

The space surrounding the infant's microenvironment should ensure auditory, visual, and physical privacy for the infant–parent dyad. In addition, the space must comfortably ensure parental presence without impinging on the work-space area necessary to deliver safe, quality care (White, Smith, & Shepley, 2013).

The aesthetics of the care environs coupled with the space attributes impacts the individuals who work and interact within that setting. Art, aesthetics, and space are the fundamental components of a welcoming, healing environment and convey respect for human dignity. Ranging from lighting strategies to the use of color, incorporating nature, utilizing various flooring materials and sound-absorbing materials, single-patient room design, displaying visual art, the use of ambient and focal music, and feng shui—elements of space and environment create an atmosphere that inherently affects health for both the patient and the clinician (Schweitzer et al., 2004; Ulrich, 1997, 2001).

The Human Environment

A collaborative health care team that emanates teamwork, mindfulness, and caring	1. Collaboration—Interprofessional rounds occur weekly and ensure consistency in care across all disciplines 2. Caring—Direct care providers demonstrate caring behaviors that include adherence to hand hygiene protocols, cultural sensitivity, open listening skills, and a sensitive relationship orientation 3. Communication—Verbal, written, and behavioral (nonverbal) communication is respectful, complete, and patient centered

So never lose an opportunity of urging a practical beginning, however small,
for it is wonderful how often in such matters the mustard-seed germinates and
roots itself.—Florence Nightingale

The human environment for age-appropriate care is comprised of the following elements: (a) communication—verbal, written, behavioral; (b) caring—self-care, transpersonal care, relationship-based care; and (c) collaboration—reconciliation, respect, mutual intent. These three essentials create a foundation of trust and teamwork with a shared vision of healing and patient safety.

Communication is a fundamental requisite for all human encounters and the one in which we struggle with most in health care. How do we communicate with our colleagues? How do we communicate with parents? How do we communicate with our patients? Collectively, across all disciplines, we struggle to standardize communications and, in truth, avoid communication when it is difficult. The mediums we use—verbal, written, and behavioral (nonverbal)—give us a broad palette to draw upon, but, oftentimes, are insufficient to meet the communication challenges we encounter in the NICU.

Handoff communication is a high-profile communication challenge identified by The Joint Commission (TJC) with recommendations to utilize structured communication strategies such as SBAR (Situation, Background, Assessment, Recommendation) to ensure the transfer of complete and concise information. An alternative communication structure is PURE (Purposeful, Unambiguous, Respectful, and Effective), a communication strategy that has been demonstrated to be effective in ensuring quality care coordination for high-risk births as well as promoting teamwork in the perinatal setting (Gephart & Cholette, 2012; Veltman & Larison, 2007). These communication frameworks work well in controlled situations, but, as many clinicians know only too well, there is a subculture in many clinical settings that is disruptive to the exchange of vital information necessary to provide quality, safe patient care.

In 2008, TJC issued a *Sentinel Event Alert* regarding behaviors that undermine a culture of safety.

> Intimidating and disruptive behaviors can foster medical errors, contribute to poor patient satisfaction and to preventable adverse outcomes, increase the cost of care, and cause qualified clinicians, administrators and managers to seek new positions in more professional environments. Safety and quality of patient care is dependent on teamwork, communication, and a collaborative work environment. To assure quality and to promote a culture of safety, health care organizations must address the problem of behaviors that threaten the performance of the health care team. (p. 1)

Addressing these disruptive behaviors requires coordination with the elements of the human and systems environment, specifically, communication, collaboration, and accountability. Policies and procedures must be developed and supported not only by frontline professionals but also by managers and administrators. What this looks like in day-to-day practice is a collaborative effort among staff, leadership, and human resources to outline an action plan that can be implemented, evaluated, and then hardwired into the culture of care (Longo, 2010).

Beyond conversations with our peers and colleagues, NICU clinicians must communicate with parents and the tiny infants they care for in the NICU. One of the biggest challenges clinicians have in parental communications is consistency of information. Nurse–parent communication must reflect partnership with parents and convey reassurance and support (Jones, Woodhouse, & Rowe, 2007). This approach empowers, educates, and validates the role of the parent. Brett et al. (2011) present a systematic mapping review of effective communication interventions with parents of preterm infants. This kind of insightful information informs the NICU clinicians on how to best facilitate communication with parents and ensure optimal exchange of critical information.

Communication with the infant is often a secondary activity related to a care interaction. Historically, the introduction of an impending care encounter between the hospitalized infant and a NICU clinician would be abrupt, mediated by the infant's care schedule and additional procedural requirements. The clinician would enter the microenvironment of the infant, reposition the infant to gain access for assessment, begin the care proceedings, complete the care actions, reposition the infant, and then terminate the care encounter by closing portholes of the incubator, often with minimal verbal exchange. Ideally, this was done quickly and expediently so that the infant could return to a restful state. To put these actions in the context of an adult care encounter is commensurate with the nurse entering the patient's room without knocking or introducing self, removing the bed linens and lifting up the patient's hospital gown to gain access for a physical examination, returning the gown and bed linens to their original position, and then leaving the patient's room, all without saying a word. Adults are able to put these types of care events in context and, even though this is not a desired care interaction, these types of scenarios do happen in the hospital setting. For neonates with poor visual acuity and who spend most of their time in a sleep state, this type of abrupt introduction to a care interaction is neither respectful nor age appropriate. Based on an understanding of the developmental and physiological needs of the infant, it is recommended that the clinical team create some type of greeting or introduction to the infant of an impending care interaction and initiate the introduction when the infant is in a wakeful or aroused state. In doing this, the clinician providing age-appropriate care frames the care event and consequently manages the associated stress of the care encounter by acknowledging the personhood of the infant.

> *Act so that you treat humanity, whether in your own person or in that of another, always as an end and never as a means only.*—Kant

The caring elements of the human environment encompass self-care, transpersonal care, and relationship-based care. These are quintessential components of professional nursing practice. Self-care in nursing is often overlooked but is truly crucial in the delivery of quality care. The act of caring for others is a giving act and can often deplete an individual's internal reserve.

> In preparation for takeoff, flight attendants review the safety protocol with passengers and inform them: should cabin pressure change, an oxygen mask will be released from the compartment above their seat. Flight attendants request that passengers place the oxygen mask on self first, before helping others.

This is analogous to self-care in nursing; before helping others the nurse must ensure that she is in a healthy state, and put her oxygen mask on first, before helping others.

Making time for true relaxation—not just time off from work—but authentic quiet time by oneself, is essential. Nursing is so people-oriented and other-focused that time alone is often not seen as valuable. Yet, alone-time can become a practice that enhances self-caring.—Duffy

Transpersonal caring and relationship-based caring combine to reflect the therapeutic use of self in human interactions driven by our relationships with peers, colleagues, patients, and their families. This healing presence is reflected in attentiveness, listening, teaching, and technical competence (Godkin, 2001).

Transpersonal, relationship-based caring encounters with patients and their families allow us to share the human experience of suffering; to bear witness to and validate the patient's experience; and through authentic presence, manage and mitigate the distress associated with the patient's current reality (Koloroutis, 2004; Naef, 2006; Watson, 2005).

Transpersonal and relationship-based caring with colleagues is vital not only for effective teamwork but for patient safety as well. To quote Henry Ford, "Coming together is a beginning. Keeping together is progress. Working together is success."

In addition to a multigenerational nursing workforce, neonatal nursing is part of an interprofessional, multidisciplinary team. Integrating the diverse psychosociocultural and spiritual characteristics of the team into the culture of care of the NICU is both challenging and stimulating, creating opportunities for growth through collaboration. Despite these opportunities, however, attitudes and interpersonal dynamics can compromise effective teamwork, quality care delivery, patient safety, and staff satisfaction.

Caring for each other and establishing collaborative relationships begin with the nurse. As Duffy (2009) states,

> Nurses set the tone on patient care units and can "make or break" other healthcare providers as they try to deliver care...Taking the responsibility to ensure a safe and private place to practice and creating a culture of teamwork are caring behaviors that fall within the realm of professional nursing.

Power dynamics and trust impact interprofessional collaboration (McDonald, Jayasuriya, & Harris, 2012). Effective patient-oriented teams committed to the delivery of evidence-based, age-appropriate care in the NICU must address and resolve these interpersonal challenges. Trust is the cornerstone for successful collaboration and develops over time with good communication. The human dimension of the healing environment is foundational in changing the NICU culture to provide consistently reliable, trauma-informed age-appropriate care.

The Systems Environment

Evidence-based policies, procedures, and resources are available to sustain the healing environment over time	1. Standards—Core measures for age-appropriate care provide the standard of care for all patient-care encounters 2. Resources—Both human and material resources to support the implementation of age-appropriate care are in place 3. Accountability—All staff hold themselves and their colleagues accountable for the provision of evidence-based, age-appropriate care

Standards, resources, and accountability make up the systems' environment for age-appropriate care. Standards are evidence-based best practices in the delivery of age-appropriate care (Coughlin, 2011). Resources are human as well as materials and products necessary to operationalize the standards. Accountability is being responsible for one's actions and one's adherence to clearly communicated performance expectations. Accountability begins at the frontline but extends to the boardroom.

Standardization, resource utilization, and accountability create the personality or the culture of an organization; consistency, trustworthiness, and empowerment are critical for effective organizational leadership (Kane-Urrabazo, 2006). Elements of the systems environment are intertwined with human dimensions. Achieving a culture of accountability to evidence-based standards is greater than the number of policies, procedures, and protocols.

The goal of the systems environment is to establish reliability in the delivery of evidence-based, trauma-informed age-appropriate care. High reliability is a function of technical competence, collaboration, communication, leadership, and process design (Parrotta, Riley, & Meredith, 2012). In presenting the evidence for trauma-informed care in the NICU and subsequently outlining evidence-based best practices to mitigate trauma and deliver age-appropriate care, the NICU clinician is compelled to deliver this new standard of care.

NICU clinicians generally perceive that the tenets of developmental care are already a standard in their NICU. The expectation for the provision of a standard of care is that it is *always* provided. One example is hand hygiene compliance, an expression of caring for the patient and a hospital standard of care. It is unacceptable for a clinician to comply

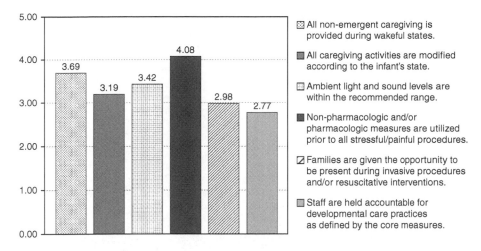

Figure 6.1 *Frequency of providing age-appropriate care in the NICU.*

with hand hygiene protocol sometimes, often, or never. Compliance is expected *always*, with every patient encounter. Now, this being said, hospitals struggle with hand hygiene compliance, despite it being the single most effective strategy to reduce the risk of a hospital-acquired infection. This same struggle exists with the provision of age-appropriate care. In a random survey of NICU clinicians regarding the frequency in which they deliver age-appropriate care ranging from *never* (0) to *always* (5), the average response hovered between sometimes and often (Figure 6.1).

The systems attribute of the healing environment must have the courage and commitment to demand high reliability in meeting evidence-based standards of performance. The right thing must be done every time, for every infant, and by every clinician in the provision of trauma-informed age-appropriate care.

eLearning modules for the Healing Environment can be accessed at the Quality Caring Institute Moodle site. Go to moodle.caringessentials.org and select the course titled "Transformative Nursing in the NICU."

CHAPTER 7: *Protected Sleep*

WHAT IS PROTECTED SLEEP IN THE NICU?

Outlined in the original paper and restated in the recent National Association of Neonatal Nurses (NANN) guidelines, the core measure for protected sleep encompasses the assessment of sleep–wake states, supporting sleep throughout the hospital stay, and educating families about sleep safety in the hospital and at home (Coughlin, 2011; Coughlin, Gibbins, & Hoath, 2009). Table 7.1 outlines the attributes and criteria for this very important core measure for age-appropriate care.

Why Is Sleep Important for the Premature and Critically Ill Infant?

Sleep plays a critical role in cognitive, psychomotor, and temperament development (Ednick et al., 2009). Sleep has also been linked with immune function enhancement and modulation of the hypothalamic–pituitary–adrenal (HPA) axis with a reduction of stress hormones, as well as an increase in growth hormone (GH) and prolactin (Besedovsky, Lange, & Born, 2012; Ganz, 2012). Well-organized sleep cycling is associated with autonomic stability and stable oxygenation in preterm infants (Lehtonen & Martin, 2004; Ludington-Hoe et al., 2006). Consolidation and maturation of sleep–wake patterns are associated with enhanced language learning skills as well as higher scores on the Mental Developmental Index (MDI) of the Bayley Scales for Infant Development at 6 months of age (Dionne et al., 2011; Gertner et al., 2002).

During fetal development, the fetus exhibits periods of activity and quiescence, which gradually give way to more structured cycles of rest and activity as neural circuitry unfolds and evolves (Peirano & Algarín, 2007). By 25 to 30 weeks gestation, sleep and sleep cycles begin to emerge;

Table 7.1 *Attributes and Criteria for Protected Sleep in the NICU*

Attribute	Criteria
Infant sleep–wake states will be assessed, documented, and will guide all nonemergent care interactions	1. All nonemergent caregiving is provided during wakeful states
	2. Sleep–wake states are assessed and documented
	3. Scheduled caregiving is contingent on the infant's sleep–wake state and adapted accordingly
Care strategies that support sleep are individualized for each infant and documented	1. Caregiving activities that promote sleep (i.e., containment, swaddled bathing, massage/Yakson, skin-to-skin care) are integrated into the patient's daily plan of care
	2. All caregiving activities are modified according to the infant's state
	3. Sensory environment is maintained within recommended ranges, and cycled lighting to support nocturnal sleep is implemented appropriately
Families are educated on the importance of sleep safety in the hospital and the home	1. Family education on caregiving activities that promote safe sleep is provided
	2. Parenting opportunities are provided and supported to promote infant sleep
	3. Staff role model "Back to Sleep" practices for families once the infant has demonstrated postural integrity in supine position or has reached 40 weeks corrected gestational age

these two processes are essential for sensory system development, brain plasticity, and long-term memory and learning (Graven & Browne, 2008b; Scher, Johnson, & Holditch-Davis, 2005). The emergence of distinct sleep states, active sleep (AS) and quiet sleep (QS), has been correlated with central nervous system maturation and each state corresponds with distinct neuronal activity that is requisite for optimal physiologic and developmental integrity (Peirano, Algarín, & Uauy, 2003).

Weisman et al. (2011) observed sleep state transitions in a cohort of low birth weight (BW) preterm infants (mean BW 1,500 g; mean gestational age [GA] 31 weeks). Three state transition patterns emerged without any differences observed in BW, GA, or medical risk among the study participants. Infants with state transitions represented by shifts between QS and wakefulness (as opposed to AS, cry or active, and QS) demonstrated greater neuromaturation, less negative emotionality, better cognitive development, and better verbal, symbolic, and executive competence at 5 years of age (Figure 7.1).

Consequences of Sleep Deprivation in the Premature and Critically Ill Infant

Sleep deprivation studies have demonstrated that both rapid eye movement (REM) sleep and non-REM (NREM) sleep impact experience-dependent neural plasticity; in animal studies of REM sleep deprivation (AS equivalent for infants) the subjects had reduced cerebral cortex and brainstem volumes (smaller brains) than controls (Tarullo, Balsam, & Fifer, 2011).

Optimal immune function requires a balance between cell-mediated immunity and humoral immunity. Sleep deprivation disrupts this balance with a shift toward cell-mediated immunity; this imbalance compromises immune function and results in significant clinical implications for the critically ill individual (Ganz, 2012). In addition, studies have shown that, following vaccination, sleep-deprived subjects had a twofold decrease in antigen–antibody-specific titers (Besedovsky et al., 2012).

Extrapolating consequences based on the research associated with optimal sleep, one can deduce that sleep deprivation in this highly vulnerable patient population will also compromise growth, emotion regulation, language, and learning as well as executive functioning.

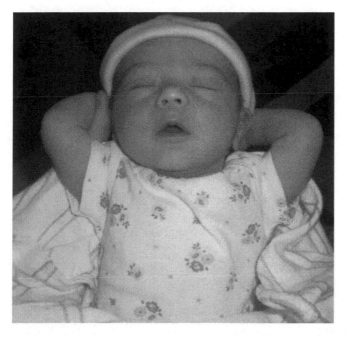

Figure 7.1 *Quiet sleep state.*

Table 7.2 *Age-Related Sleep Needs*

Average Daily Sleep Needs per Age	
Premature infants (less than 37 weeks)	17–20 hr/day
Newborn to 2 months old	12–18 hr/day
3 months to 1 year old	14–15 hr/day

Table 7.3 *Sleep–Wake State Descriptions of Preterm Infants*

Active sleep	Eyes closed; respirations uneven; sporadic motor movements with low muscle tone between movements; intermittent rapid eye movement (REM)
Quiet sleep	Eyes closed; respirations regular and abdominal in nature; tonic motor tone; motor activity limited to occasional startles or sighs

Neonatal sleep organization is a prerequisite for optimal neuroma-turation, physiologic stability, and psychoemotional and cognitive integrity. Promoting and protecting sleep in the neonatal intensive care unit (NICU) is crucial. Although all infants admitted to the NICU are neonates, their age-specific sleep requirements may not be the same and evolve over the hospital stay. The neonate of 25 weeks GA does not have the same sleep needs as the critically ill term infant or the infant born at 30 weeks gestation who has been hospitalized for 2 months. Providing age-appropriate protected sleep must be individualized and reflect a knowledge of sleep needs of infants over the first year of life (Table 7.2).

EVIDENCE-BASED CARE STRATEGIES FOR PROTECTED SLEEP

Assessment of Sleep–Wake States

Infant behaviors, including sleep–wake states, guide nursing care interactions. In addition, these behaviors change over time, as the infant matures. Although much more has been known about full-term sleep–wake behaviors, understanding these behavior patterns in premature infants has required significantly more investigation. Early studies of human fetal motility laid the foundation for understanding movement and behavior in premature individuals. These studies have demonstrated that fetal behaviors become more organized as gestation progresses (Arduini et al., 1986; De Vries & Fong, 2006; Nijhuis, Prechtl, Martin, & Bots, 1982). Working from this base of knowledge, Holditch-Davis and Edwards (1998) were able to define two sleep states in a cohort of high-risk preterm infants (Table 7.3).

Building off this work, Holditch-Davis, Scher, Schwartz, and Hudson-Barr (2004), in a longitudinal descriptive study of 134 preterm infants with BWs less than 1,500 g, confirm that sleep–wake behaviors mature over time and the frequency of sleep–wake transitions increases through 40 weeks corrected GA and then begins to decrease after 43 weeks. At term, sleep cycles of 50 to 60 minutes are contrasted to the sleep cycle of the preterm infant, which equals 75 minutes; in addition, the proportion of AS to total sleep time at 34 weeks is about 60%, decreasing to 50% at term, and to 25% at 6 months of age (Heraghty, Hilliard, Henderson, & Fleming, 2008; Scher et al., 2005). This important information highlights the need for age-appropriate care competence for the NICU clinician in protecting and promoting sleep across the continuum of individuals cared for in the NICU.

The assessment of the infant's sleep–wake state should guide non-emergent clinical care activities to prevent or at least minimize sleep fragmentation and sleep deprivation. Figure 7.2 represents the Neonatal Sleep Wake Assessment Tool© Caring Essentials Collaborative, LLC. This teaching tool helps neonatal clinicians learn sleep behaviors associated with AS and QS (Figure 7.3) and use this information to guide care delivery.

Transitioning to an age-appropriate care delivery model requires patience, creativity, teamwork, and support. The NICU clinician is confronted with a myriad of competing priorities; providing individualized, age-appropriate patient-centered care in this setting can be challenging.

> *The majority of infants in the newborn ICU are placed on a scheduled routine; it may be 8–11–2–5, 9–12–3–6, or some other variation of scheduled times for care interactions. This schedule allows the clinician to ensure that he or she completes all the tasks necessary to provide safe, clinical care during the hospital stay. More often than not, these scheduled routines do not align with the infant's biobehavioral clock. Practicing age-appropriate care requires a balance between completing the tasks on our checklist and respecting the developmental human needs of the individuals we serve.*

Indicator	0	1	2	Total
Eyes	Lids closed with intermittent rapid eye movement (REM)	Lids closed; no REM observed	Lids open	
Respiration	Uneven respirations	Relatively regular and abdominal	Regular respirations; may be crying	
Facial Expression	Negative facial expressions (cry face or a frown)	Quiet facies; occasional startle or sigh	Interactive facies	
Motor Activity	Sporadic motor movements, muscle tone low between movements	Tonic level of motor tone is maintained and motor activity is limited to startles and sighs	Motor activity varies but is usually high	
			Cumulative Score	

Figure 7.2 *Neonatal Sleep Wake Assessment Tool.*

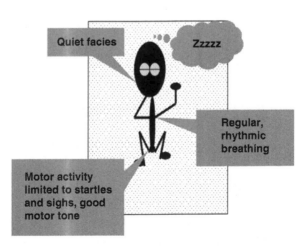

Figure 7.3 *Quiet sleep.*

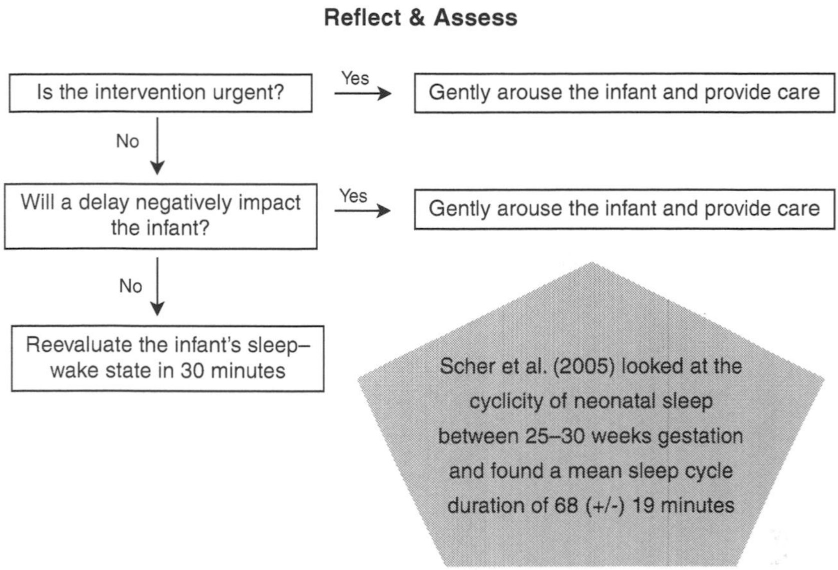

Reflect & Assess

Figure 7.4 *Suggested algorithms for waking infant for care activity.*

Figure 7.4 outlines a suggested algorithm to reflect and assess if the infant should be awakened from sleep in order to provide nonemergent care.

Supporting Sleep in the NICU

Supporting sleep for the hospitalized infant is achieved through environmental modifications and caregiving interactivities (Allen, 2012). The sleep–wake cycle is organized around homeostatic and circadian processes. Circadian rhythmicity is linked to light–dark cycles and the suprachiasmatic nucleus plays a prominent role in setting the biological clock (Duffy & Czeisler, 2009; Heraghty et al., 2008). Cycled lighting in the hospital nursery for premature infants more than or equal to 32 weeks of age induces distinct patterns of rest–activity that persist beyond discharge (Rivkees, Mayes, Jacob, & Gross, 2004). As the neonate advances in age and requires hospitalization beyond the neonatal period (the first 28 days of life), supporting the changing rest–activity patterns with daytime naps can be facilitated with minor adaptations to the ambient light environment.

Variability in the lighting needs of the diverse patient populations served in the NICU can be a logistical challenge. If possible, cohorting infants based on their age-related lighting needs might optimize the quality and quantity of their sleep.

Sound levels conducive to sleep range between 30 and 35 dB. Average sound levels in the NICU can range from 52 dB to as high as 117 dB (Brown, 2009; Peixoto, de Araújo, Kakehashi, & Pinheiro, 2011; Pinheiro, Guinsburg, Nabuco, & Kakehashi, 2011). In addition, noise levels inside the incubator can range between 45 and 79 dB and are influenced by the ambient noise levels in the NICU (Pinheiro et al., 2011). The single most significant contributor to the sound environment is the staff. To understand how these sound levels compare to everyday familiar sounds, please refer to Figure 7.5.

Sounds	dB(A)
Rocket launching	180
Jet engine, gunshot	140
Thunderclap	130
Jet take-off (threshold for pain)	120
Rock concert, car horn	110
Firecracker, subway train	100
Heavy truck, lawnmower, blender	90
Alarm clock, hair dryer	80
Noisy restaurant, business office	70
Normal conversation	60
Light traffic, average home	50
Living room, quiet office	40
Library, soft whisper	30
Rustling leaves	20
Threshold for sound	0

Figure 7.5 *Various sound levels.*

Effective strategies to reduce the sound have been described in Chapter 5 and are requisite to protect sleep in the premature and critically ill, hospitalized infant.

Kangaroo care (KC), also known as skin-to-skin care, has been demonstrated in numerous studies to facilitate bonding, improve autonomic stability, promote thermoregulation, and impact the maturation of sleep architecture (Engler et al., 2002; Feldman, Weller, Sirota, & Eidelman, 2002; Jeffries & Canadian Paediatric Society, Fetus and Newborn Committee, 2012; Ludington-Hoe et al., 2006; Nyqvist et al., 2010; Scher et al., 2009). The data supporting this practice strategy as an effective intervention to promote and support sleep is highlighted in the work of Ludington-Hoe et al. (2006) and Scher et al. (2009), who present the first research linking skin-to-skin/KC to neurophysiologic correlates.

Despite the supportive research, however, clinicians struggle to implement KC in the neonatal critical care setting. Barriers to implementation include concerns about safety, especially for infants with high acuity (Engler et al., 2002). Hendricks-Muñoz et al. (2013) revealed possible sociocultural factors that were barriers to KC in the NICU from their prospective cohort design study of neonatal nurses and mothers of preterm infants. Using an anonymous, self-report questionnaire, the researchers discovered discrepancies in nurse perceptions of the role of parental presence in the NICU (21% of nurses vs. 67% mothers strongly agreed that parents should be encouraged to be present in the NICU). More than 60% of the nurse respondents agreed that KC benefits the infant; however, the majority of nurses felt that time spent in KC should be limited and that this type of parent–infant interaction should not be provided daily.

Although education and confidence building in the skills required to facilitate KC safely in the NICU are necessary, there appear to be additional opportunities to explore the barriers to this practice strategy. NICU nurses committed to providing age-appropriate care will identify and resolve these barriers with creative, respectful, and safe solutions to consistently and reliably provide evidence-based, patient-centered KC.

Infant massage, swaddling, gentle touch, and Yakson therapy also are soothing sensual experiences that can facilitate sleep for the premature and critically ill, hospitalized infant. Cortisol, a byproduct of HPA axis activation, inhibits sleep. As presented in Chapter 2, stress is a reality for infants hospitalized in the NICU, and this stress, in addition to other environmental influences, can contribute to sleep fragmentation and sleep deprivation (Buckley & Schatzberg, 2005; Ganz, 2012). Infant massage and other tactile therapies have been documented to reduce neurochemical and hormonal markers of stress; Smith et al. (2013), in a randomized longitudinal study, were able to demonstrate the positive and lasting effects of massage on medically stable preterm infants (29–32 weeks GA) using heart rate variability as a marker of autonomic nervous system (ANS) reactivity or stress tolerance. Massaged infants in this study demonstrated improved ANS functional development, which may improve their ability to maintain healthy sleep–wake cycles.

In an earlier study on the effect of massage on weight gain and sleep, Dieter, Field, Hernandez-Reif, Emory, and Redzepi (2003) were able to demonstrate a statistically significant increase in weight gain after 5 days of massage therapy as well as note that infant sleep patterns appeared to be more organized with fewer hours spent in sleep and more time in quiet and active alert states. Massage therapy appears to reduce stress, improve weight gain, and increase the infant's capacity for engagement with caregivers and the environment.

Gentle healing touch (the act of placing one hand on the infant's head and the other hand placed on the infant's abdomen) and Yakson (gentle caressing of the body) have both demonstrated the capacity to calm and soothe a premature, hospitalized infant, increase sleep states, reduce stress level and energy expenditure, and decrease oxygen dependency during the early hospitalized period (Bahman Bijari, Iranmanesh, Eshghi, & Baneshi, 2012).

The application of music therapy (MT) in the NICU has been studied extensively over the past decade; a recent meta-analysis confirms significant benefits of MT on heart rate, behavior state, oxygen saturation, sucking/feeding ability, and length of stay (Standley, 2012). Gilad and Arnon (2010) describe additional benefits to live music and singing in the NICU, including enhanced weight gain, a decrease in stress indicators, and an observed sense of humanity in the intensive care environment.

As the name implies, MT is a deliberate intervention of soothing sounds to promote optimal physiological and psychological responses from the listener. MT is *not* the radio playing in the background; it is *not* a tape recording or MP3 recording of white noise, storytelling, nursery rhymes, or any other type of audio stimulus playing within the microenvironment of the infant. These examples are simple variations of noise, which has been demonstrated to negatively affect sleep state and sleep quality in preterm infants (Wachman & Lahav, 2011).

In addition to live music and singing, several scientists have examined the use of maternal biological sounds as a form of MT in the NICU.

Loewy, Stewart, Dassler, Telsey, and Homel (2013), in a randomized mul-
tisite trial of 272 premature infants aged 32 weeks gestation or older,
examined the effect of three live music interventions on infant vital
sign parameters, feeding and sleep. Outcomes revealed that the use of
informed, intentional live sound and parent-preferred lullabies benefited
the infants across the selected dimensions with statistical significance
observed in sleep behaviors (p <.001). Doheny, Morey, Ringer, and Lahav
(2012) also noted a decrease in the incidence of apnea and bradycardia in
preterm infants exposed to maternal voice and heart beat; understanding
the link between breathing and sleep, the efficacy of MT for sleep quality
is validated in Doheny's study (Lehtonen & Martin, 2004).

The dosing of MT as biological maternal sounds and the implication
of this intervention for the NICU nurse were evaluated by Zimmerman,
Keunen, Norton, and Lahav (2013) and uncovered the need to support the NICU nurse in the adoption of this new practice intervention.
Empowering the bedside clinician to use clinical judgment, grounded by
the nurse's relationship with the infant, improved utilization of this effective, evidence-based strategy.

Parent Partnerships and Education for Safe Sleep

NICU admission is terrifying not only to the infant but also to the parents. Joseph, Mackley, Davis, Spear, and Locke (2007) looked at components of perceived stress of fathers of surgical NICU infants using the
Parent Stressor Scale (PSS) and discovered paternal stress was highest in
the domains of parental role alterations and infant appearance.

In a qualitative study of parental perspectives on neonatal intensive
care, Pepper, Rempel, Austin, Ceci, and Hendson (2012) uncovered the
importance of parent relationships with clinicians and the parents' desire
for the clinician to provide hope and facilitate understanding of the situation as well as validate their parental role. Parents expect and need
caregivers to care authentically and communicate regularly about their
infant's medical, surgical, and human needs and support the emerging
role of the parent (Guillaume et al., 2013).

Protecting, promoting, and supporting sleep is the perfect role for the
NICU parent. In partnering with parents in the NICU, the parent role is
validated by providing basic care, comfort, and support to their hospitalized infant. Building confidence and competence is part of the shared
journey for all parents, but is presented with unique challenges in the
NICU.

Education, mentoring, and role modeling by NICU clinicians facilitate the successful transition of the parent from novice to expert in supporting safe sleep for their infant (Grazel, Phalen, & Polomano, 2010).

Gelfer, Cameron, Masters, and Kennedy (2013) utilized a quality improvement methodology to translate the American Academy of Pediatrics (AAP) guidelines for safe sleep practices into NICU nursing practice. Using an algorithm outlining when to start safe sleep practice, educating staff nurses, and placing reminders at the bedside, the group was able to increase "back to sleep" practices with statistical significance ($p < .001$) as well as increase parental compliance with home safe sleep practices postdischarge from 23% to 82%.

SUMMARY

Protecting sleep in the NICU is everyone's responsibility. Ensuring the environment is conducive to sleep through noise reduction and appropriate lighting, incorporating best practices that support and promote sleep, and partnering with parents in the provision of these evidence-based strategies will positively improve the quality of sleep for this incredibly vulnerable and susceptible patient population.

Interactivity for sleep assessment can be accessed at the Quality Caring Institute Moodle site. Go to moodle.caringessentials.org and select the course titled "Transformative Nursing in the NICU."

CHAPTER 8: *Age-Appropriate Activities of Daily Living*

WHAT ARE AGE-APPROPRIATE ACTIVITIES OF DAILY LIVING?

Age-appropriate activities of daily living (ADLs) include postural support, alimentation, and skin care management (Coughlin, 2011; Coughlin, Gibbins, & Hoath, 2009). Table 8.1 outlines the attributes and criteria for this core measure set.

Why Are Age-Appropriate ADLs Important for the Premature and Critically Ill Infant in the Neonatal Intensive Care Unit (NICU)?

Age-appropriate ADLs are the everyday life tasks, independent of disease, that human beings participate in for personal care and include eating, bathing, dressing, toileting, and repositioning self. Functionally dependent on others for these daily activities, infants learn trust, empathy, and attachment through the task relationship. We are wired to be social, beginning in utero (Castiello et al., 2010), and ADLs provide the stage in which the developing human learns the dance of social interactions and relationships with an adult caregiver. It is through intersubjectivity, interpersonal relations, and, yes, the mirror neuron system that infants learn about the world and their place in it (Allen & Williams, 2011; Bastiaansen, Thioux, & Keysers, 2009; Fogel, de Koeyer, Bellagamba, & Bell, 2002; Gallese, 2003).

ADL activities are important for the premature and critically ill infant not only for the psychological and socioemotional dimensions associated with shared caring interactions (Gibbins, Hoath, Coughlin, Gibbins, & Franck, 2008; Korsch, 1978) but also the physical implications. Preserving

Table 8.1 *Age-Appropriate ADLs in the NICU*

Attribute	Criteria
Age-appropriate postural alignment is documented to provide comfort and safety, physiologic stability, and support optimal neuromotor development	1. Each infant is positioned and handled to support age-appropriate postural integrity during all caregiving activities
	2. Infant position is evaluated with every infant interaction and modified to support postural alignment and integrity
	3. Positioning aids are gradually removed and "back to sleep" and "tummy to play" practices are implemented as the infant demonstrates physiologic flexion of the upper body in supine position and/or reaches 44 weeks corrected gestational age
Age-appropriate alimentation will be infant-driven, individualized, nurturing, functional, and developmentally appropriate to ensure safety	1. Nonnutritive sucking is offered with each nonoral feeding contingent on the infant's state
	2. Assessment of feeding readiness cues and the quality of the oral feeding is documented with each oral feeding encounter
	3. Education regarding the benefits of breast milk is provided and family feeding choice is supported
Age-appropriate skin integrity is documented to ensure assessment, protection, and care	1. Preterm infants are bathed no more frequently than every 3 days; term infants are bathed based on their individual needs; pH-neutral cleanser is used
	2. Skin integrity, including mucous membranes, is assessed using a reliable assessment tool at least once per shift and documented (Braden Q Scale or similar tool)
	3. The skin surface and mucous membranes are protected during application, utilization, and removal of adhesive products and other medical devices

and protecting musculoskeletal, gastrointestinal, and integumentary function is crucial to the short- and long-term health outcomes of the premature and critically ill infant.

Humanizing these routine care activities in the NICU is critical and creates an opportunity for NICU clinicians to partner with the infant–parent dyad in the provision of ADLs. This partnership cultivates parental confidence and competence and validates the parental role while meeting the fundamental, age-appropriate needs of the infant.

In the absence of parental presence, however, the NICU clinician providing age-appropriate care is responsible for ensuring that the human caring dimensions of these routine care activities are provided.

Mindfulness, presence, and authentic caring are crucial aspects of age-appropriate ADLs in the NICU (Jarrín, 2012; Siegel, 2010).

Consequences Associated With an Absence
of Age-Appropriate ADLs in the NICU

The physiological ramifications of not providing age-appropriate ADLs in the NICU include (a) compromised musculoskeletal development, including flexor and extensor abnormalities, postural deformities, and delayed attainment of developmental milestones; (b) alimentation challenges, including oral aversion and long-standing issues regarding feeding, nutrition, and growth; and (c) skin integrity compromise, resulting in pain, possible scarring, and increased risk of infection.

Consequences from a psychological perspective correspond to the relational experience between infant and caregiver associated with ADLs. Emotions are shared through motor, somatosensory, and affective simulations mediated by neural circuits of the mirror neuron system and subcortical structures, including the amygdala, hypothalamus, hippocampus, and orbitofrontal cortex (Bastiaansen et al., 2009; Decety, 2010). Accordingly, if the task relationship does not convey empathy, or is unpleasant or aversive, these early experiences associated with social interaction jeopardize future relationships, emotion regulation, and physical and mental health (Als et al., 2004; Decety, 2010; Low & Schweinhardt, 2012; Niwa, Matsumoto, Mouri, Ozaki, & Nabeshima, 2011).

EVIDENCE-BASED CARE STRATEGIES
THAT SUPPORT AGE-APPROPRIATE ADLs

The evidence-based care strategies across all age-appropriate ADLs are predicated on the assumption the clinician exhibits mindfulness and authentic presence during the task relationship. The relational nature of infant care interactions is exemplified by the clinician's capacity to read and interpret the infant's biobehavioral cues and use this feedback to adapt and modify the care interaction. Stress and readiness cues represent the vocabulary of the premature and critically ill infant. It is incumbent on the caregiver to "listen" and share in the dialogue with the infant as care tasks unfold (Davidson & McEwen, 2012; Fogel et al., 2002; Nummenmaa et al., 2012).

Postural Support

Age-appropriate postural alignment is documented to provide comfort, safety, and physiologic stability, and support optimal neuromotor development	1. Each infant is positioned and handled to support age-appropriate postural integrity during all caregiving activities
	2. Infant position is evaluated with every infant interaction and modified to support age-appropriate postural alignment and developmental progression
	3. Positioning aids are gradually removed and Back to Sleep and Tummy to Play practices are implemented as the infant demonstrates physiologic flexion of the upper body in supine position and/or reaches 44 weeks corrected gestational age

Age-appropriate positioning and postural integrity for the neonatal patient population are mediated by the infant's chronology and medical/surgical limitations. The postural needs of the infant born at 25 weeks gestation are different from the term infant hospitalized for a diaphragmatic hernia. In addition, as the hospital stay extends beyond the neonatal period (the first 28 days of extrauterine life), NICU clinicians must be competent in supporting the progression of gross motor development over the first year of life. Facilitating this developmental progression requires a multidisciplinary team approach, collaboration, and partnership with parents to minimize developmental delay and optimize outcomes.

The ultimate goal of gross motor development over the first year of life is for independent movement and freedom of the infant to use his or her hands to explore and learn about the world (Gerber, Wilks, & Erdie-Lalena, 2010). De Vries and Fong (2006), in their thorough overview of normal fetal motility, describe the onset of specific movement patterns observed in the fetus and the implications of these movement patterns postdelivery under the influence of the force of gravity. Understanding the impact of gravity on movement and the musculoskeletal system has clinical implications for the NICU nurse.

Flexor tone develops in a caudad-cephalad progression, with lower extremity flexion beginning around 29 to 32 weeks and arm flexion beginning at 35 to 37 weeks (Allen & Capute, 1990; Sweeney & Gutierrez, 2002). Evidence supports the need for supportive positioning to reduce abnormalities associated with the force of gravity and musculoskeletal vulnerability during hospitalization. Routine changes in position, while ensuring postural alignment, preserve neuromuscular and osteoarticular function in low-risk preterm infants (Vaivre-Douret, Ennouri, Jrad, Garrec, & Papiernik, 2004). The influence of gravity on the underdeveloped musculoskeletal system of the premature infant results in flattened posture and external rotation of the hips and shoulder retractions, and forces lateral rotation of the head/neck (Clarac, Vinay, Cazalets, Fady, & Jamon, 1998; Morningstar, Pettibon, Schlappi, Schlappi, & Ireland, 2005; Vaivre-Douret et al., 2004). In addition, cranial deformations secondary to the force of gravity and infant severity of illness limiting spontaneous movement plague this vulnerable patient population. Dolichocephaly in the preterm infant and plagiocephaly in the term infant impact brain morphology and possibly influence brain function and neurodevelopmental integrity (Collett et al., 2012; McManus & Capistran, 2008; Mewes et al., 2007).

Forced lateral rotation of the head and neck in the premature infant, either induced by the influence of gravity or related to infant position (i.e., prone, supine), has been associated with changes in cerebral hemodynamics (Pellicer, Gayá, Madero, Quero, & Cabañas, 2002; Pichler, van Boetzelar, Müller, & Urlesberger, 2001; Malusky & Donze, 2011). Accordingly, Limperopoulos et al. (2008) reported fluctuations in cerebral dynamics of preterm infants during routine caregiving, including minor manipulations (auscultation), diaper changes, endotracheal (ET) tube suctioning, ET tube repositioning, and complex events; circulatory changes were associated with cranial ultrasound parenchymal abnormalities. Ancora et al. (2010) looked at brain hemodynamics and posture in a cohort of medically stable preterm infants with gestational age (GA) less than 30 weeks. Using near-infrared spectroscopy, the authors found that cerebral blood volume was decreased in stable preterm infants with GA less than or equal to 26 weeks during head rotation. Fluctuations in cerebral blood flow and immature autoregulatory capacity in premature infants are associated with an increased risk for intraventricular hemorrhage and parenchymal injury (Ballabh, 2010; Limperopoulos et al., 2008).

Midline, neutral head position in infants less than 32 weeks gestation for the first 72 hours of life is a best-practice recommendation (Ancora et al., 2010; Malusky & Donze, 2011), with implications to continue to support a midline orientation until the infant attains hemodynamic stability (Chock, Ramamoorthy, & Van Meurs, 2012). Age-appropriate postural support during routine caregiving has been shown to reduce stress behaviors in preterm infants (Comaru & Miura, 2009; Grenier, Bigsby, Vergara, & Lester, 2003; Liaw, Yang, Chou, Yang, & Chao, 2012). Postural support at rest for premature infants that facilitates spontaneous, antigravity movement, hip flexion, and shoulder adduction increases bone mineralization in very low birth weight (VLBW) infants, promotes age-appropriate postural orientation, and promotes neuromaturation (Aucott, Donohue, Atkins, & Allen, 2002; Eliakim, Nemet, Friedland, Dolfin, & Regev, 2002; Ferrari et al., 2007).

For the term and postterm infant, postural support should correspond to the infant's developmental motor stage and medical liabilities/limitations (e.g., a term infant who may be sedated and require neuromuscular blockade will benefit from supportive positional aids versus the term infant with typical motor tone who is spontaneously moving).

Recommendations for best practice for postural support (Sweeney & Gutierrez, 2010):

- Optimize alignment: neutral neck–trunk; semiflexed, midline extremity posture; neutral foot alignment.
- Support posture and movement within "containment boundaries" of rolls, swaddling blankets, or other positioning aids; avoid creating an immobilization barrier.
- Modify positioning and handling to promote regulation of behavioral states that enhance short-duration interaction and sleep states that promote growth.
- Offer positions that allow controlled, individualized exposure to proprioceptive, tactile, visual, or auditory stimuli; monitor for signs of behavioral stress from potential overstimulation.

Assessment and documentation of postural alignment inform the NICU clinician of the infant's medical limitations in postural support as well as the understanding of what works and what does not work for the infant from a comfort perspective, based on infant biobehavioral responses to various positioning strategies. The Infant Position Assessment Tool (IPAT) was developed as an educational resource for NICU clinicians with a goal of standardizing developmentally supportive positioning for premature infants. Coughlin, Lohman, and Gibbins (2010) created and subsequently evaluated the tool in conjunction with a systemwide education program focused on developmentally supportive care in a Level-III NICU setting, and were able to demonstrate an increase in the frequency in which infants were positioned supportively as defined by the IPAT. Standardization of postural goals for premature and critically ill infants ensures consistency and reliability in the provision of evidence-based best practices in postural support.

The implementation of the American Academy of Pediatrics (AAP) guidelines for safe sleep in the NICU can be a challenge. NICU clinicians struggle to find the balance between prone positioning routines of the hospitalized infant and transitioning the infant to a supine sleep position in preparation for discharge (McMullen, 2013). NICU clinicians are influential role models and educate parents through their actions. Standardizing NICU practices regarding safe sleep strategies will promote postdischarge supine sleep position for NICU graduates (Gelfer, Cameron, Masters, & Kennedy, 2013; Grazel, Phalen, & Polomano, 2010; McMullen, Lipke, & LeMura, 2009).

Between 2 and 4 months of age, newborns should be supported in building strength through their shoulder girdle. This can be facilitated by positioning the infant prone to play, and assists the infant in meeting this early gross motor milestone (Gerber et al., 2010; Sweeney & Gutierrez, 2002). Opportunities for tummy time include kangaroo care as well as supervised periods when the infant is in prone position.

Alimentation

Age-appropriate alimentation will be infant-driven, individualized, nurturing, functional, and developmentally appropriate to ensure safety	1. Nonnutritive sucking is offered with each nonoral feeding contingent on the infant's state
	2. Assessment of feeding readiness cues and the quality of the oral feeding is documented with each oral feeding encounter
	3. Education regarding the benefits of breast milk is provided and family feeding choice is supported

The process of giving or receiving nourishment is alimentation, and this concept embraces not only oral feeding but enteral and parenteral nutrition as well. Premature and critically ill infants require optimal nutrition to survive. NICU clinicians struggle to meet the dietary requirements of this vulnerable population while preserving those aspects of alimentation that extend beyond mere sustenance and embrace the sociosensual dimensions of alimentation.

Feeding is fun, social, and something many of us embrace without a lot of focus on the nutritional aspects of what we are ingesting. Age-appropriate alimentation in the NICU is a combination of optimal caloric intake and an optimal feeding experience.

What does it look like in the NICU? For the infant who is given nothing by mouth (NPO), it is offering nonnutritive sucking, providing opportunities for kangaroo care to facilitate infant exploration of the maternal landscape, and providing exposure to positive olfactory input relative to feeding (i.e., maternal scent, breast milk; Fucile, McFarland, Gisel, & Lau, 2012; Lipchock, Reed, & Mennella, 2011; Pimenta et al., 2008); for the infant receiving enteral tube feedings, it is nonnutritive sucking and being held during the feeding infusion (Fucile et al., 2012; Pimenta et al., 2008); and for the infant transitioning from gavage feeding to oral feeding (breast or bottle), it is ensuring the feeding experience is driven by the infant, determined by feeding readiness behaviors (Jones, 2012; Lau, Geddes, Mizuno, & Schaal, 2012; Ludwig & Waitzman, 2007; Nye, 2008; Pickler, 2004; Ross & Philbin, 2011).

Assessment of feeding readiness cues is framed by an understanding of the maturational processes associated with suck, swallow, and respiration coordination (Barlow, 2009). Gewolb and Vice (2006) completed an elegant evaluation of these maturational changes and demonstrated that while suck and swallow rhythms stabilized before 36 weeks, the coordination with respiration occurs closer to term. Combining an understanding of developmental feeding physiology and infant feeding cues plays a crucial role in feeding success. Changing the feeding goal from a volume focus to a quality of experience focus results in earlier attainment of full oral feedings in preterm infants (Kirk, Alder, & King, 2007; Newland, L'huillier, & Petrey, 2013).

Breast-feeding is the gold standard for alimentation in newborns, with particularly significant benefits for prematurely born individuals, including decreased incidence in feeding intolerance, nosocomial infection, necrotizing enterocolitis, chronic lung disease, developmental delay, and rehospitalization post-NICU discharge (Meier, Engstrom, Patel, Jegier, & Bruns, 2010). Dougherty and Luther (2008) developed a "birth to breast" feeding care map for use in the NICU. The authors created a user-friendly visual algorithm, based on the infant's corrected GA and postnatal age, to guide feeding progression based on motor, state, and respiratory support dimensions.

Evidence-based best practices that support age-appropriate alimentation in the NICU focus on positive oral experiences, infant-driven engagement in feeding interactions, education for parents on the benefits of breast milk, and encouraging and supporting breast-feeding in the NICU (Meier et al., 2010).

Skin Care Management

Age-appropriate skin integrity is documented to ensure assessment, protection, and care	1. Preterm infants are bathed no more frequently than every 3 days; term infants are bathed based on their individual needs; a pH-neutral cleanser is used
	2. Skin integrity, including mucous membranes, is assessed using a reliable assessment tool at least once per shift and documented (Braden Q Scale or similar tool)
	3. The skin surface and mucous membranes are protected during application, utilization, and removal of adhesive products and other medical devices

Skin is a complex, multifunctional organ that arises from the same embryonic germ layer as the central nervous system and is the interface that separates self from the environment (Hoath & Narendran, 2001). Skin integrity is vital for survival and highlighted by the multiple tasks it performs immediately after birth, including barrier function to minimize transepidermal water loss, thermoregulation, infection control, immune surveillance, acid mantle formation, antioxidant function, protection from ultraviolet (UV) light, tactile discrimination, and attraction to caregiver (Hoath & Narendran, 2001; Telofski, Morello, Mack Correa, & Stamatas, 2012). Preserving the integrity of these functions lies in the ability of the NICU clinician to employ prevention strategies that respect the vulnerability and majesty of the integumentary system.

Barrier function is incomplete in preterm infants and places this patient population in a precarious position relative to their intensive care needs. With frequent invasive procedures from intubations to vascular access, skin and mucous membrane integrity is threatened. Functional skin maturity is reached by 34 weeks gestation; however, postnatally, skin matures rapidly, even in very preterm infants, and reaches functional maturity at the surface layer within 2 to 8 weeks postnatal age (Ness, Davis, & Carey, 2013). Despite this accelerated maturation, premature skin remains fragile and warrants vigilance in protective maintenance.

Protective strategies include a judicious, evidence-based approach to cleansing and preserving skin integrity. Immersion bathing has demonstrated less heat loss as opposed to sponge bathing, which can compromise vagal tone in preterm infants (Lee, 2002; Ness et al., 2013). Frequency of bathing neonates should be minimized and a pH-neutral cleanser is preferred over plain water (Blume-Peytavi, Hauser, Stamatas, Pathirana, & Garcia Bartels, 2012; Ness et al., 2012). Quinn, Newton, and Pieuch (2005), in a randomized clinical trial, demonstrated the safety of every 4th-day bathing for preterm infants.

Pressure ulcer and skin breakdown are hospital-acquired complications that are preventable through routine assessment and implementation of evidence-based prevention measures. The Neonatal Skin Condition Scale (AWHONN, 2007) has demonstrated validity and reliability as an effective assessment tool for use in the NICU (Lund & Osborne, 2004). In addition, the Braden Q Scale, a valid and reliable tool designed for pressure ulcer risk assessment in pediatric patient populations, has clinical implications for the NICU clinician (Noonan, Quigley, & Curley, 2011).

The majority of infants hospitalized in the NICU require adhesive applications to affix and secure various medical devices necessary to manage the infant's medical or surgical condition. Minimizing the application of adhesives to ensure safety but reduce associated complications of dermal stripping, pain, and noxious sensory stimulation is requisite for the clinician providing age-appropriate care. The use of hydrocolloid adhesives is preferred to reduce skin injury and bonding agents should be eliminated from the armamentarium of dressing supplies (Ness et al., 2012). Mineral oil or other petroleum-based products may be effective in removing stubborn adhesives when warm water does not work, but the area should be cleansed following removal of the adhesive, as these agents can be absorbed through the skin, posing an additional health risk (Ness et al., 2012).

SUMMARY

Providing age-appropriate ADLs in the NICU is vital for physiological and psychological wellness for the premature and critically ill infant. Ensuring postural integrity, safe and sensual alimentation, and protecting skin integrity through relationship-oriented interactions validate the personhood of the infant and elevate the professional practice of neonatal nursing.

---

eLearning modules for ADLs can be accessed at the Quality Caring Institute Moodle site. Go to moodle.caringessentials.org and select the course titled "Transformative Nursing in the NICU."

CHAPTER 9: *Prevention and Management of Pain and Stress*

WHAT IS PAIN AND STRESS PREVENTION AND MANAGEMENT IN THE NICU?

Pain and stress prevention and management in the neonatal intensive care unit (NICU) are commitments to minimizing and mitigating noxious and distressing consequences associated with hospitalization and critical illness. This includes not only a proactive approach to managing the pain and stress associated with necessary invasive procedures but also critically reviewing the necessity of various painful procedures often considered routine in an intensive care environment (e.g., routine labs, scheduled feeding tube changes, dressing changes, etc.).

Outlined in the original paper and restated in the recent National Association of Neonatal Nurses (NANN) guidelines, this core measure focused on assessment and management of pain and stress during NICU hospitalization (Coughlin, 2011; Coughlin, Gibbins, & Hoath, 2009). In this chapter you will be introduced to a revision of this core measure emphasizing the prevention of pain and stress in the NICU as well as ensuring the routine assessment and management of pain and stress throughout the NICU stay.

Table 9.1 outlines the attributes and criteria for this very important core measure.

Why Are Pain and Stress Prevention and Management Important for the Premature and Hospitalized Infant?

The neuroanatomical and neuroendocrine mechanisms that facilitate the transmission of a painful stimulus are functional in the fetus at 20 to

Table 9.1 *Attributes and Criteria for Pain and Stress Prevention and Management in the NICU*

Attribute	Criteria
Prevention of pain and stress is an expressed goal in the daily management of the hospitalized infant	1. Potentially painful and/or stressful daily care activities are critically reviewed and revised as to their clinical necessity based on the infant's current status
	2. Noninvasive technologies will be employed over invasive technologies to gather necessary biological data
	3. A pain and stress prevention policy is in operation and reviewed regularly with staff (minimum annually)
Pain and/or stress is assessed and managed before, during, and after all procedures until the infant returns to his or her baseline level of comfort; interventions and infant responses to stress-relieving and pain-management interventions are documented	1. A valid, age-appropriate pain assessment tool is utilized for routine interactions as well as anticipated painful procedures
	2. Pain and stress assessments guide all caregiving activities, and these activities are adapted based on infant feedback to minimize pain and stress
	3. Nonpharmacologic and/or pharmacologic measures are utilized prior to all stressful and/or painful procedures; infant response to these interventions is documented and guides future management strategies
Family is involved and informed of the pain and stress management plan of care for their infant(s); involvement and information sharing is documented	1. Parents are involved and informed of the pain and stress management plan of care for their hospitalized infant(s)
	2. Family education regarding infant pain and stress cues is provided
	3. Family is encouraged, empowered, and supported to provide comfort to their infant

22 weeks gestation (Bellieni, 2012; Canadian Pediatrics Society, 2000; Loizzo, Loizzo, & Capasso, 2009; Puchalski & Hummel, 2002). In fact, Johnston, Fernandes, and Campbell-Yeo (2011) explain that premature individuals, due to heightened sensitivity and a broader neuronal receptive field for nociceptive input, may also perceive nonnoxious stimuli as painful (such as gentle touch or the feel of clothing over the affected area); this hypersensitivity is complicated by delayed maturation of the descending pain pathways that modulate the pain experience—consequently, preterm infants may have a prolonged experience of pain (Bhutta & Anand, 2002).

When pain is prolonged and unmanaged or undermanaged, the neonate's response is to decrease energy expenditure and he or she

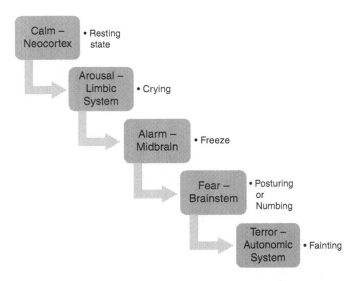

Figure 9.1 *Acute response to threat.*

enters a state of passivity, decreasing heart and respiratory rate, and decreasing oxygen consumption (American Academy of Pediatrics [AAP], 2006). Perry, Pollard, Blakely, Baker, and Vigilante (1995) liken these observations to the acute response to threat, whereby increasing threat alters mental state, from calm to arousal, alarm to fear, and then terror.

As the threat intensifies, the neural mediators of the response regress from the level of the neocortex to the limbic system, the midbrain, the brainstem, and finally the autonomic system (Figure 9.1). Unmanaged or undermanaged pain and stress are perceived and actual threats to the premature and critically ill infant.

To exemplify this, I share a story from my clinical past:

> *I was asked to start an IV on a very small infant after several of my colleagues had made unsuccessful attempts. As I came upon the infant's bedside, I found the infant lying supine on the incubator tray, which was pulled out to facilitate access to the infant. There was a warming light over the infant and an IV cart nearby. The infant's extremities were extended and limp, her head turned to one side, and eyes closed. I asked my colleague if I should come back at another time and she implored me to make an attempt, as the infant had been without IV fluid for a while and had "fallen asleep" during the last IV attempt.*

In fact, the infant had not fallen asleep: the infant essentially disassociated from the experience due to the profound stress and threatening nature of the interaction. In an attempt to preserve her physiologic integrity, with her hypothalamic–pituitary–adrenal (HPA) axis in a state of hyperactivation, the more primitive structures of her central nervous system, specifically her brainstem and autonomic nervous system, took over in an effort to reduce her oxygen consumption and energy expenditure associated with the unmanaged stress and pain of this invasive procedure.

With repeated exposures to painful experiences, the infant can develop a hyperalgesia or an increased responsiveness to a painful stimulus, even develop allodynia or a pain response to a nonpainful stimulus (AAP, 2006).

Given that pain is a stressful experience, Smith et al. (2011), using the Neonatal Infant Stressor Scale (NISS; Newnham, Inder, & Milgrom, 2009), were able to demonstrate regional alterations in brain structure and function related to the exposure of stressors during the NICU. The NISS (see Appendix) creates a systematic way of assessing and subsequently managing stressful events in the NICU. This tool provides clinicians with a standard reference guide depicting the myriad of procedures and care activities that warrant pain and stress prevention and management.

In two prospective studies designed to understand epidemiology and management of neonatal pain, researchers have revealed that, despite advances in knowledge in the vulnerability of premature and critically ill infants to pain, we still hurt babies. Despite clinicians' awareness that most NICU procedures are painful, only one third of infants undergoing a painful procedure receive appropriate pain management, and premedication for known painful procedures occurred in less than half of the infants (Simons et al., 2003). Carbajal et al. (2008) looked at a cohort of 430 infants with a mean gestational age of 33 weeks over the first 14 days of hospitalization and prospectively collected data on all stressful or painful procedures performed, along with corresponding pain management strategies. The researchers report that of the 14,413 painful procedures observed, 79% of the procedures were performed without any specific pharmacological or nonpharmacological intervention.

Consequences Associated With Unmanaged or Undermanaged Pain and Stress in This Vulnerable Population

All stress may not be pain but all pain does activate a stress response. Unmanaged or undermanaged pain not only impacts neural circuitry related to nociception but also causes regional cerebral hemodynamic changes, as well as induces HPA axis activation and alterations that impact pain and stress responses over the life span (Bartocci, Bergqvist, Lagercrantz, & Anand, 2006; Grunau, Weinberg, & Whitfield, 2004; Puchalski & Hummel, 2002).

Chronic pain experiences during infancy increase the risk for childhood sleep problems, difficulties in self-regulation, attention and learning disorders, as well as lifelong alterations in pain perception and chronic pain syndromes in adulthood (Karr-Morse & Wiley, 2012; Low & Schweinhardt, 2012). Beggs, Currie, Salter, Fitzgerald, and Walker (2012) highlight the impact of neonatal pain experiences on adult pain perceptions. Neonatal pain, neonatal surgery, and tissue injury prime the neuroimmune response, altering nociceptive pathways and increasing pain sensitivity in later childhood and adulthood (Beggs et al., 2012; Fitzgerald & Walker, 2009; Peters et al., 2005).

Adverse, traumatizing experiences in early life (such as prematurity and neonatal critical illness requiring intensive care) have been linked with psychiatric pathologies as well as stress-induced physiological dysfunction, both of which impact long-term health outcomes and the global burden of disease associated with neonatal intensive care (Grunau et al., 2005; Johnstone et al., 2011; Konturek, Brzozowski, & Konturek, 2011; Lai & Huang, 2011; National Scientific Council on the Developing Child, 2005; Pechtel & Pizzagalli, 2011). Unmanaged and undermanaged pain and stress in the NICU are traumatic experiences. It is a moral imperative for neonatal clinicians to prevent, assess, and manage pain and stress in the vulnerable individuals served in the newborn ICU.

Barriers

Despite this moral imperative, however, challenges and barriers exist in the consistently reliable prevention, assessment, and management of stress and pain in the premature and critically ill infant patient population. Byrd, Gonzales, and Parsons (2009) identified a knowledge–practice gap in their descriptive survey study of a cohort of California neonatal nurses. While more than 90% of the nurse respondents acknowledged that newborns experienced more pain than older children and that it is a key responsibility of the nurse to prevent and manage pain, only 45% of the nurses agreed that their unit managed newborn pain well.

Latimer, Johnston, Ritchie, Clarke, and Gilin (2009), using a cross-sectional research design, looked at factors affecting the provision of evidence-based procedural pain management strategies in two Canadian tertiary care centers. Their findings point to the level of nurse–physician collaboration and nursing work assignments as key predictive factors. Similar to Byrd et al. (2009), the Latimer team exposed that nurses' knowledge of pain and pain protocols were not predictors for the implementation of evidence-based procedural pain management.

EVIDENCE-BASED CARING STRATEGIES TO PREVENT, ASSESS, AND MANAGE PAIN AND STRESS IN THE NICU

Prevention of pain and stress is an expressed goal in the daily management of the hospitalized infant	1. Potentially painful and/or stressful daily care activities are critically reviewed and revised as to their clinical necessity based on the infant's current status
	2. Noninvasive technologies will be employed over invasive technologies to gather necessary biological data
	3. A pain and stress prevention policy is in operation and reviewed regularly with staff (minimum annually)

Prevention of pain and stress in the NICU is a challenge due to the nature of critical illness. Understanding the deleterious effects of pain and stress on the developing brain, the NICU nurse is poised as advocate and champion to the premature and critically ill infant. Routine caregiving is stressful and sometimes painful and requires a thoughtful, individualized approach to care. Many NICU nurses employ a clustered care approach to the provision of routine care; for example, if the infant is scheduled for routine assessment at 8 a.m., in addition to the assessment, other care activities are "clustered" together during the assessment. Clustered care that focuses on completing the tasks at the expense of the infants is painful and stressful and does not reflect the principles of trauma-informed age-appropriate care.

Holsti, Grunau, Whifield, Oberlander, and Lindh (2006) discovered that infants experienced heightened arousal and disorganization during clustered care and highlight the importance of a cue-based individualized approach to care. A cue-based approach requires attunement on the part of the clinician to read the nonverbal, biobehavioral responses of the infant as the care interactivity unfolds. The clinician then uses these cues to continue, pause for recovery, or discontinue the care interaction with the infant. Clustered care must be a balance between meeting the task completion needs of the clinician and the infant's needs to maintain homeostasis.

Blood sampling is the most frequently occurring painful and stressful procedure in the NICU, with infants undergoing between 1 and 21 heel punctures or venipunctures per day (Kapellou, 2011). A judicious review of routine lab draws must be part of the daily plan of care. Oftentimes, infants undergo frequent and painful blood sampling with little impact to their daily medical management. Utilizing noninvasive, nonpainful methods of biological data collection must be incorporated into the culture of care in the NICU. When a blood draw is clinically indicated, venipuncture has demonstrated fewer biobehavioral pain responses than heel stick (Ogawa et al., 2005; Shah, Taddio, Bennett, & Speidel, 1997).

The use of noninvasive technologies should be employed to reduce neonatal exposure to pain and stress. Pulse oximetry, pulse CO-oximetry, transcutaneous blood gas monitoring, and transcutaneous bilirubinometry are a few of the available technologies (Carceller-Blanchard, Cousineau, & Delvin, 2009; Jung et al., 2013; Sandberg, Brynjarsson, & Hjalmarson, 2011).

The NANN has recently published their third edition *of Newborn Pain Assessment and Management Guidelines for Practice* (Walden & Gibbins, 2012). When developing a pain and stress prevention policy for your NICU, these guidelines provide evidence-based recommendations and rationale for nursing practice and care of the hospitalized preterm and term neonate.

Pain and/or stress is assessed and managed before, during, and after all procedures until the infant returns to his/her baseline level of comfort; interventions and infant responses to stress-relieving and pain-management interventions are documented	1. A valid, age-appropriate pain assessment tool is utilized for routine interactions as well as anticipated painful procedures
	2. Pain and stress assessments guide all caregiving activities, and these activities are adapted based on infant feedback to minimize pain and stress
	3. Nonpharmacologic and/or pharmacologic measures are utilized prior to all stressful and/or painful procedures; infant response to these interventions is documented and guides future management strategies

Pain assessment and management are the cornerstone for high-quality, trauma-informed age-appropriate care in the NICU and are mandated by The Joint Commission (TJC) for hospital accreditation. Pain is a subjective, unpleasant sensory and emotional experience with actual or potential tissue injury. The challenge of accurately and sensitively assessing pain in premature and critically ill infants lies is their inability to verbalize the experience. The preverbal state of this vulnerable population in no way diminishes their experience and, as was presented earlier, they are at risk for heightened experience of pain due to their developmental immaturity.

Neonatal pain assessment tools must be multidimensional and demonstrate reliability and validity as well as feasibility in the clinical setting (Duhn & Medves, 2004). The multidimensionality of the tool enables the clinician to ensure comprehensive and accurate assessment of information and includes physiological as well as behavioral parameters (e.g., facial activity and body movements). Near-infrared spectroscopy and EEG techniques to monitor neonatal pain responses at the cortical level offer new hope for the effective validation of neonatal pain assessment tools and technologies (Holsti, Grunau, & Shany, 2011).

Once the appropriate tool has been identified for use in the NICU, this, in and of itself, does not mean that neonatal pain is effectively managed (Franck & Bruce, 2009). The assessment and identification of a neonatal pain experience require prompt, effective treatment (Lago et al., 2009). It is not enough to document the pain assessment score; there must be an intervening action. NICU clinicians must collaborate and obtain consensus in outlining a pain management plan of care.

Management strategies for pain and stress include both pharmacological as well as nonpharmacologic interventions. Pharmacological interventions include the use of opioids, benzodiazepines, barbiturates, chloral hydrate, propofol, and acetaminophen and topical anesthetics, all of which present some degree of hazard to the premature and critically ill infant (Whit Hall, 2012). Topical anesthetics have not proven effective in heel sticks, venipunctures, or IV insertions (Johnston et al., 2011; Larsson et al., 1996; Lehr & Taddio, 2007).

The efficacy of nonpharmacologic strategies has been extensively studied in the neonatal patient population and includes sensory stimulation interventions, nutritive solutions, and maternal interventions (Fernandes, Campbell-Yeo, & Johnston, 2011; Johnston et al., 2011). Gitto et al. (2012) were able to demonstrate that a combination of fentanyl administration (opiate) and sensory saturation provided superior analgesia in preterm infants experiencing procedural pain. Sensory saturation is a strategy to engage the infant across several sensory pathways to distract the central nervous system from interpreting the pain sensation. Sensory saturation is an important nonpharmacological treatment strategy but must be monitored, using a cue-based approach to avoid overstimulating the infant.

Containment and postural supportive strategies (facilitated tuck and swaddling) provide proprioceptive, tactile, and vestibular stimulation;

when combined with nonnutritive sucking, they reduce infant pain scores and promote biobehavioral stability (Cignacco et al., 2012; Johnston et al., 2011; Liaw et al., 2012). The additive effect of oral sucrose with non-nutritive sucking and facilitated tucking not only provided pain relief during heel stick but also facilitated the infant's transition back to sleep postprocedure (Cignacco et al., 2012; Liaw et al., 2013). Naughton (2013) compiled an integrative review and concludes that the combined use of sucrose and nonnutritive sucking is a safe, effective, and clinically significant intervention to relieve procedural pain in both preterm and term infants.

In addition to procedural pain associated with blood sampling, pain and distress associated with endotracheal intubation have been studied, and it has been demonstrated that the use of premedication significantly improves intubating conditions, decreases time and number of attempts to perform intubation, and minimizes intubation-related trauma to the airway (AAP, 2006; Carbajal, Eble, & Anand, 2007; Kumar, Denson, & Mancuso, 2010). The most current recommendation from the AAP is that, except for emergent intubations, newborns should be premedicated for endotracheal intubation (Kumar et al., 2010).

Tracheal suctioning, feeding tube insertion, and retinopathy of prematurity (ROP) examinations have been associated with biobehavioral markers of pain. There remains significant variability in the management of stress and pain associated with these common NICU patient experiences as well as the management of states of illness, such as the infant requiring mechanical ventilation. As best practice in the management of the mechanically ventilated infant remains controversial, NICU clinicians are charged with being vigilant and responsive to these infants' comfort needs and exploring safe, effective therapies (Kaneyasu, 2012; McPherson, 2012; Menon & McIntosh, 2008).

Tracheal suctioning has demonstrated disturbances in cerebral hemodynamics in addition to biobehavioral pain responses (Axelin, Salanterä, & Lehtonen, 2006; Kaiser, Gauss, & Williams, 2008). Facilitated tucking by parents as well as employing a four-handed care model (where one clinician provides support, containment, and reassurance as the other clinician performs the suctioning procedure) during both of these nonpharmacologic interventions resulted in a reduction of stress and defense behaviors (Axelin et al., 2006; Cone, Pickler, Grap, McGrath, & Wiley, 2013).

Nasal insertion of a feeding tube is painful, inducing a pain response similar to a heel stick. In a randomized, double-blind, placebo-controlled trial, McCullough, Halton, Mowbray, and Macfarlane (2008) were able to demonstrate the efficacy and safety of a single dose of sublingual 24% sucrose in reducing the biobehavioral pain responses associated with nasal insertion of a neonatal feeding tube. In a subsequent study (Kristoffersen, Skogvoll, & Hafström, 2011), the researchers were able to demonstrate that the combination of a pacifier with a concentrated sucrose solution reduced the pain score by more than 50%.

Samra and McGrath (2009), in a systematic review of pain management strategies employed during ROP examinations, concluded that despite a general consensus that this procedure is painful, pain management remains inadequate. This highlights the previously discussed challenges in implementing pain prevention and pain management practices in the NICU. Bedside clinicians, clinical and administrative leadership, as well as organizations and accrediting bodies must resolve these inequities of care to our most vulnerable members of society.

Unmanaged pain *must* become a "never event" for the premature and critically ill, hospitalized infant. Parents as partners in care are perfectly positioned to advocate for and facilitate effective pain prevention interventions in the NICU.

Family is involved and informed of the pain and stress management plan of care for their infant(s); involvement and information sharing is documented	1. Parents are involved and informed of the pain and stress management plan of care for their hospitalized infant(s)
	2. Family education regarding infant pain and stress cues is provided
	3. Family is encouraged, empowered, and supported to provide comfort to their infant

Family involvement in the comfort of their infant is a requisite for healthy parent–infant development. Although no parent wants his or her newborn to experience pain, when pain is a reality due to life-threatening illness and intensive care hospitalization, parents must be armed with knowledge about their infant's pain experience and pain behaviors as well as effective evidence-based pain management strategies.

Parent involvement in pain management of their hospitalized infant was recently investigated by Franck et al. (2011) in a randomized, controlled trial and, although parent stress during the NICU stay was not impacted, parental role attainment and increased satisfaction in caregiving in the early postdischarge period were positively affected. An additional finding that warrants further investigation was the observed increase in nursing pain assessment documentation in the intervention group. Parental involvement in pain management may provide nurses with a visual reminder for improved pain assessment practices.

Parental involvement in pain management is also recommended as a best-practice strategy in the third edition of the NANN *Newborn Pain Assessment and Management Guideline for Practice* (2012). The role of parents in neonatal pain management is a relatively new concept for NICU clinicians. An exploration of parents' perceptions and feelings about partnering with clinicians to manage the pain experience of their infant validates their desire to actively advocate for and comfort their infant (Franck, Oulton, & Bruce, 2012).

Educating, empowering, and partnering with NICU parents are key components of family-centered care. Factors affecting parental presence include parental involvement in providing comfort and care for their infant (Heinemann, Hellström-Westas, & Hedberg Nyqvist, 2013). Knowledge about pain prevention, assessment, and management engages parents and validates the parental role.

Maternal-driven, nonpharmacological pain management strategies have been well documented and include skin-to-skin care, breast-feeding, and maternal auditory and olfactory sensory stimulation (Campbell-Yeo, Fernandes, & Johnston, 2011). The challenge in accessing these effective therapies lies in creating an environment conducive to parental presence and participation in the NICU (Blomqvist, Frölund, Rubertsson, & Nyqvist, 2013; Greisen et al., 2009; Heinemann et al., 2013).

SUMMARY

The consistently reliable prevention, assessment, and management of pain and stress in the NICU are core requirements in providing trauma-informed age-appropriate care.

---

eLearning modules for pain and stress prevention, assessment, and management can be accessed at the Quality Caring Institute Moodle site. Go to moodle. caringessentials.org and select the course titled "Transformative Nursing in the NICU."

APPENDIX: NEONATAL INFANT STRESSOR SCALE

INSTRUCTIONS: Enter the time that the procedure was performed (eg: 9:15 am)

Name: _____

Date: _____

Acute Items						Chronic Items	
extremely stressful (score 5)		7am–9am	9am–11am	11am–1pm	1pm–3pm	**extremely stressful** (score 5)	
Multiple attempts inserting IV, IA, UAC/UVC							
Intubation							
Insertion pneumothorax chest drain							
Eye examination							
very stressful (score 4)						**very stressful** (score 4)	
Suctioning of ETT tube						having asystemic infection	
Suctioning of nose and mouth						HFO/Jet vent without sedation	
Removing infant from incubator/bed (unwrapped)							
Insertion of IV, IA, UAC/UVC							
Insertion of percutaneous long line							
Insertion of nasal CPAP tube							
Lumbar puncture							
Surgery							
Heel pricks							
moderately stressful (score 3)						**moderately stressful** (score 3)	
Nappy changes						nursed in radiant warmer	
Position changes						local infection	
Removal of IV						HFO/Jet vent with sedation	
Receiving nasal CPAP						Hudson Prong CPAP	
Insertion of Hudson Prong						fasting for surgery	
Insertion of nasogastric tube						recovering from surgery	
Gavage feed						pneumothorax chest drain	
Removing infant from incubator/bed (wrapped)						conventional ventilation w/o sedation	
Cardiac echocardiogram							
Ultrasound							
CT/MRI							
X-ray							
Being weighed							
a little stressful (score 2)						**a little stressful** (score 2)	
Mouth care						nursed in incubator	
Eye toilet						IV fluids	
IV Flushing (to ensure IV patency)						IV/IA/UAC/UVC in situ	
Sampling eg. blood gases						conventional ventilation with sedation	
Removal of UAC/UVC						lumber puncture recovery	
Stomach aspiration via NGT						intranasal oxygen	
ECG						head box oxygen	
Attachment of monitor sensors						nasogastric tube in situ	
Application of cream to body						phototherapy	
TOTAL ACUTE STRESS SCORE						**TOTAL CHRONIC STRESS SCORE**	

Reprinted with permission from Elsevier Publishers.

CHAPTER 10: *Family-Centered Care*

WHAT IS FAMILY-CENTERED CARE IN THE NICU?

A consensus on the definition of family-centered care (FCC) remains elusive, although it has been recognized as a necessary element in the neonatal intensive care unit (NICU; Gooding et al., 2011; Kuo et al., 2012; Thomson, Moran, Axelin, Dykes, & Flacking, 2013). Despite the lack of consensus, the Institute for Family-Centered Care has put forth four key concepts of FCC: dignity and respect, information sharing, participation, and collaboration. Johnson, Abraham, and Shelton (2009) highlight the link between patient and FCC and quality and patient safety. These concepts and perspectives frame trauma-informed FCC.

Trauma-informed FCC in the NICU is a commitment to protecting and preserving the integrity of the family in crisis, ensuring optimal infant–parent attachment and parental role development to promote short-term and long-term family integrity.

The FCC core measure attributes and criteria presented in this chapter are revised from the previous publications (Coughlin, 2011; Coughlin, Gibbins, & Hoath, 2009).

Table 10.1 outlines the latest evidence-based attributes and criteria for this very important core measure.

Table 10.1 *Attributes and Criteria for FCC in the NICU*

Attribute	Criteria
Family has 24-hour unrestricted access to their infant and is supported in role-validating activities during the NICU stay	1. Family is a valued partner of the health care team and is encouraged to participate in family rounds and change of shift report
	2. Family is encouraged to be present during invasive and resuscitative procedures
	3. Family is empowered and supported in relationship and role-validating activities with their infant, including (but not limited to) routine infant cares, feeding activities, and other parenting interactions
The family's level of emotional well-being and parental confidence and competence is assessed and documented weekly	1. Mental health professionals resource families weekly and as necessary
	2. Family observations and input regarding their infant's well-being, behavioral cues, and preferences are sought by the clinical care providers
	3. Health care providers share unbiased information regarding the medical progress of the infant weekly with the family
The family has access to resources and supports that assist them in short- and long-term parenting, decision making, and mental well-being	1. Families are invited to participate in a NICU family support group or community family support resources
	2. Culturally sensitive family education on infant safety and infant care is available in various formats
	3. Resources for the educational, social, spiritual, and financial needs of families are available

Why Is FCC Important for the Premature and Critically Ill, Hospitalized Infant?

I sustain myself with the love of family.—Maya Angelou

Developing humans require more than custodial care; they require closeness, reassurance, safety, and love (Bystrova et al., 2009; Douglas, 2010; Flacking et al., 2012; Marco, Macrì, & Laviola, 2011). Parental presence and parent partnerships in the NICU are key to optimizing outcomes for these fragile individuals across physiological, neurobiological, and psychoemotional domains (Flacking et al., 2012; Fryers & Brugha, 2013; Schore, 2001a).

I'd like to share a story of when I worked as a staff nurse on the night shift back in the early 1990s:

I was taking care of an incredibly sick, extremely premature, and growth-restricted infant. Although I've forgotten her name, I remember how frighteningly sick she was and how she was not responding to maximal life support therapies; 100% FiO₂, on the oscillator with maximum vaso-pressor support, we were losing her. Her parents never left her bedside and had never held her because she was so sick we were afraid she would not tolerate the experience. It became apparent there was nothing left we could do to save her and so we decided we would let the parents hold her before she passed away. Cautiously and gingerly my colleagues and I transferred this tiny, dying, intubated infant to her mother's bare chest. Once she was positioned safely and comfortably we put a warm blanket around baby and mother, made sure dad was OK, and stepped away to give the family some privacy. I checked in on them every so often to make sure they were OK, and after about 30 minutes I noticed that the baby's oxygen saturations (sats) started coming up; I turned the oxygen down by a percent or two and left them alone a bit longer. On my next check-in, the family wished to continue holding their daughter, and I peeked at the monitors and saw the sats were still climbing and so was her blood pressure. I turned down the oxygen a bit more this time and titrated her pressor support. Within about 3 hours of lying on her mother's chest this little girl had brought her oxygen requirement from 100% to 60% and her blood pressure was improving—it became evident that this little girl had no intention of dying that night. Embraced by the one person who was literally her whole world, this tiny, critically ill indi-vidual was telling us she wanted to live; fueled by her mother's warmth, scent, sounds—love. This little girl, who was at the precipice of death just hours earlier, was showing us that it takes more than technology to keep her alive. Her parents remained at the bedside for the next 72 hours providing continuous skin-to-skin contact as the baby slowly recovered. She was discharged home a few months later.

The clinical phenomena associated with this infant's response to skin-to-skin care are substantiated in biological processes. Skin-to-skin contact facilitates oxytocin release (a potent neuropeptide), which acti-vates central oxytocinergic mechanisms in the paraventricular nucleus of the hypothalamus and its neural circuitry to influence cardiovascu-lar regulation and cerebral oxygenation (Begum et al., 2008; Pyner, 2009; Uvnäs-Moberg, 1996).

There are biological processes associated with all human phenomena that very often exert a powerful influence on physiologic and pathophysiologic events. I know many NICU nursing colleagues who have similar stories. It is in bearing witness to these profound moments that we realize our shared humanity—we know the importance of FCC for these incredibly amazing people and we honor them by meeting their age-appropriate needs day after day in the NICU.

Consequences Associated With Disruptions in FCC for This Vulnerable Population

Maternal–infant separation is a traumatic life event for the neonate and the family. For the neonate, the absence of mother initiates a stress response mediated by the hypothalamic–pituitary–adrenal (HPA) axis. As discussed in Chapter 2, the developing human is highly vulnerable and susceptible to the deleterious effects of prolonged stress across physiologic, neurobiological, and psychoemotional domains (Lai & Huang, 2011; Sourkes, 2007).

The impact of maternal–infant separation on the mother is confounded by the life-threatening nature warranting NICU hospitalization and has been linked with maternal depression and posttraumatic stress disorder (PTSD; Ballantyne, Benzies, & Trute, 2013; Bicking & Moore, 2012; Jubinville, Newburn-Cook, Hegadoren, & Lacaze-Masmonteil, 2012). Fathers have also experienced negative consequences associated with separation from infant, including acute stress disorder and PTSD (Lundqvist & Jakobsson, 2003; Shaw et al., 2009).

Parental mental health plays a crucial role in optimizing infant developmental outcomes. Disruption of family role development compromises infant attachment relationships and results in socioemotional maladjustment and psychological pathology (Benoit, 2004).

Infant–family relationships influence neurobiology and psychology for all stakeholders. As the infant needs parental contact for optimal physiological and psychoemotional development, the parents also need a meaningful relationship with their infant to establish their identity as parents.

Implementing FCC in an intensive care environment is challenging. Given the precarious nature of the critically ill infant's medical condition, it is understandable that the bedside nurse exhibits caution in sharing infant care with potentially frightened and traumatized parents (Corlett & Twycross, 2006; DeFrino, 2009; Espezel & Canam, 2003; Hendricks-Muñoz et al., 2013). However, taking this stance and disrupting family integrity incur more harm than good. NICU clinicians must develop effective communication and collaboration skills to meet the needs of the infant–family dyad in the NICU (Wigert, Dellenmark, & Bry, 2013).

EVIDENCE-BASED CARING STRATEGIES TO SUPPORT FCC IN THE NICU

Successful implementation of FCC requires a cultural transformation within the organization, reflecting values, attitudes, and policies that acknowledge the biological and socioemotional coherence of the infant–family dyad (Flacking et al., 2012; Thomson et al., 2013).

Family has 24-hour unrestricted access to their infant and is supported in role-validating activities during the NICU stay	1. Family is a valued partner of the health care team and is encouraged to participate in family rounds and change of shift report
	2. Family is encouraged to be present during invasive and resuscitative procedures
	3. Family is empowered and supported in relationship and role-validating activities with their infant, including (but not limited to) routine infant cares, feeding activities, and other parenting interactions

Many NICUs today continue to refer to parents as visitors (Cisneros, Coker, DuBuisson, Swett, & Edwards, 2003), but parents are not visitors; parents are crucial to the immediate and lifelong health, wellness, and integrity of the neonate. Family presence and participation have been linked to decreases in length of hospital stay, increased family satisfaction, improved neurobehavioral outcomes, and parental psychological well-being (Flacking et al., 2012; Forcada-Guex, Pierrehumbert, Borghini, Moessinger, & Muller-Nix, 2006; Melnyk et al., 2006; Milgrom et al., 2013).

Family participation in rounds validates the parental role while providing a vehicle for clear, complete communications regarding the infant's medical status. A family-centered rounds strategy was evaluated in a tertiary teaching NICU and was found to statistically increase parent satisfaction scores with regard to communication as well as significantly increasing collaboration and satisfaction for neonatal nurse practitioners and neonatal fellows (Voos et al., 2011).

Parental presence during invasive procedures and resuscitative activities is endorsed by the American Academy of Pediatrics (AAP) and the Society of Critical Care Medicine, and recommended by the American Heart

Association (Dingeman, Mitchell, Meyer, & Curley, 2007). Despite this support, clinicians struggle with effective implementation of this FCC practice as parents struggle with the experience (Dingeman et al., 2007; Harvey & Pattison, 2012). Curley et al. (2012), using a pre-/post-survey methodology, evaluated the impact of practice guidelines for clinicians regarding parental presence during invasive and resuscitative procedures. Survey results indicated that, along with interprofessional education, practice guidelines positively impacted clinician perceptions and practices in supporting parental presence during invasive and resuscitative interventions.

Restoring a sense of security and comfort for the infant supports his or her homeostasis and reduces unnecessary energy expenditure. This is best facilitated through parenting activities and the provision of comfort care, aiding the process of learning to parent (Skene, Franck, Curtis, & Gerrish, 2012). The effect of maternal vocalization, parent talk, and maternal biological sounds on short-term and longer term outcomes includes a decrease in biomarkers for stress, fewer episodes of feeding intolerance, and attainment of full enteral feedings sooner than controls, improved cardiorespiratory regulation, and language skill development (Caskey, Stephens, Tucker, & Vohr, 2011; Doheny, Hurwitz, Insoft, Ringer, & Lahav, 2012; Krueger et al., 2010; Seltzer, Ziegler, & Pollak, 2010; Zimmerman et al., 2012).

Breast-feeding is the gold standard for feeding newborns, especially premature and critically ill infants. The benefits of breast milk range from nutritional to immunological dimensions (Mata, 1978), as it is the one thing only the mother can do. NICU mothers should be encouraged to breast-feed, or at least provide breast milk for their baby during the hospital stay (Rossman, Kratovil, Greene, Engstrom, & Meier, 2013).

The family's level of emotional well-being and parental confidence and competence is assessed and documented weekly	1. Mental health professionals resource families weekly and as necessary
	2. Family observations and input regarding their infant's well-being, behavioral cues, and preferences are sought by the clinical care providers
	3. Health care providers share unbiased information regarding the medical progress of the infant weekly with the family

Mental well-being of the family in crisis is crucial for short- and long-term health and wellness of the infant–family dyad (Lasiuk, Comeau, & Newburn-Cook, 2013). Routine check-ins from social services and psychology professionals are a best practice for critical care environments. The use of the Postpartum Depression Scale is effective in screening mothers for postpartum depression and expediting effective intervention (Beck, 2003; McCabe et al., 2012).

"Parent as advocate" is a natural evolution of the parenting role and has significant meaning when the infant is hospitalized in a critically ill condition. In this video, parents talk about their NICU experience and the role they played in their infant's care (www.youtube.com/watch?v=BpB0IZykzdk).

Although the parents in the video expressed a positive experience regarding their roles as parent and advocate, many parents encounter barriers to parenting in the NICU. These barriers include not only the physical aspects of noise and light but also dismissive staff attitudes that jeopardize the integrity of the parent–infant dyad (Heinemann, Hellström-Westas, & Hedberg Nyqvist, 2013).

NICU parents need comprehensive compassionate and relevant education regarding the NICU, their infant's medical or surgical condition, as well as the special human needs of their infant. Once informed, parents become the NICU nurses' best ally and fount of great insight into the behavioral cues and nuances of the premature and critically ill infant.

Melnyk et al. (2006) published the results of a randomized controlled trial evaluating a NICU parent education program entitled Creating Opportunities for Parent Empowerment (COPE); mothers in the COPE program reported less stress in the NICU and less depression and anxiety at 2 months corrected infant age. In addition, the infants in the COPE program had a shorter NICU and total hospital length of stay.

Milgrom et al. (2013) evaluated the impact of a Mother–Infant Transaction Program (MITP) on early infant developmental milestones. The program teaches parents to recognize and minimize stress responses in their preterm infants. Intervention mothers exhibited more sensitivity in caring for their infant; intervention infants demonstrated less stress cues and, at 6 months of age, they performed better than controls on cognitive and language developmental profile assessments.

Pediatric interns, residents, neonatal fellows, neonatologists, and neonatal nurse practitioners represent the primary medical providers in the NICU. The diversity in communication skills, competence, and cultural awareness of these professionals can challenge effective communication with NICU parents. In a focused education intervention on the constructs of effective communication (quantity, availability, understanding, reciprocity, and empathy) with the primary medical providers in a Level-III NICU, Weiss, Goldlust, and Vaucher (2010) demonstrated an improvement in parent satisfaction with the quantity and quality of information-shared posteducation intervention.

Armed with knowledge, understanding, and insight, NICU parents are not only invaluable for their infant but also become invaluable to the health care team.

The family has access to resources and supports that assist them in short- and long-term parenting, decision making, and mental well-being	1. Families are invited to participate in a NICU family support group or community family support resources
	2. Culturally sensitive family education on infant safety and infant care is available in various formats
	3. Resources for the educational, social, spiritual, and financial needs of families are available

Many NICUs provide family support groups or are connected to community family support resources. The March of Dimes also provides NICU family support services and programs. Health care facilities, community resources, and state and national organizations can be accessed to provide culturally sensitive resources across social, spiritual, and financial domains to ensure that the infant–family dyad is adequately resourced and supported during the trauma of neonatal intensive care hospitalization.

SUMMARY

Parents must be informed of the clinical management plan for their infant to understand their infant's experience and how they, as parent and advocate, can support and comfort their infant through the hospital stay. In fully realizing their role during the NICU stay, parents are competent and confident in understanding the implications of the NICU experience on long-term health and wellness of their infant.

Trauma-informed FCC is the evidence-based best-practice strategy for premature and critically ill, hospitalized infants. NICU clinicians and administrators have the opportunity to review FCC through the lens of evidence-based best practice and devise an effective implementation strategy for measurable outcomes (Lefaiver et al., 2009).

---

eLearning modules for trauma-informed FCC can be accessed at the Quality Caring Institute Moodle site. Go to moodle.caringessentials.org and select the course titled "Transformative Nursing in the NICU."

SECTION III: *Application, Outcomes, Relevance*

CHAPTER 11: *Integrating the Core Measures for Age-Appropriate Care Into the Culture of Care: Outcomes and Lessons Learned*

CULTURAL TRANSFORMATION IN THE CLINICAL SETTING

Translating high quality evidence into improved patient outcomes is a complex process.... Comprehensive education programs...will be the most effective.—Kalassian, Dremsizov, and Angus

Transforming a culture of care requires the transfer of knowledge into clinical practice. It is not just about the knowledge; it is about taking action with the new knowledge. The majority of neonatal clinicians universally accept the precepts of age-appropriate care in the neonatal intensive care unit (NICU), and yet an extreme inconsistency persists in its adoption into clinical practice. Embracing a systematic approach to knowledge transfer and practice change is crucial for the application and integration of this practice strategy into the culture of care in the NICU.

The Pilot Project

In 2005, the neonatal leadership team at Clinique St. Vincente, Rocourt, Belgium, began their search for an evidence-based intervention that would transform the culture of care in their Level-III NICU to one that exemplified the principles and practices of developmentally supportive care. After carefully scrutinizing various options, they elected to proceed with a revolutionary approach. They chose to integrate the core measures for developmentally supportive care (Coughlin, Gibbins, & Hoath, 2009) framed by the conceptual model, the Universe of Developmental Care (UDC; Gibbins, Hoath, Coughlin, Gibbins, & Franck, 2008), into their culture of care.

The project was comprised of an initial education phase, a subsequent translational phase that utilized the model for improvement (Plan-Do-Study-Act [PDSA] methodology), and a final evaluative phase that was separated into three periods: project baseline (data collection from January 2006 through June 2007); Study Period 1: November 2007 to April 2009; and Study Period 2: May 2009 to October 2010. In addition, the project baseline and Study Period 1 groups were followed and compared at 2 years of age for neurodevelopmental outcomes. The NICAUDIT database (Belgian neonatal network registry) provided the outcome criteria for the major clinical indicators across key neonatal morbidities. The team also looked at nursing workload as well as neurodevelopmental disability at 2 years of age, using the British Association of Perinatal Medicine (BAPM) classification criteria.

The education phase was comprised of an 8-hour training day that was repeated over several days to ensure that all direct care providers received the same information. Content was presented using adult teaching principles and included didactic and interactive experiential elements. Additionally, a 2-hour teaching session was offered to all indirect care providers and ancillary staff to ensure that all individuals who interfaced with the NICU understood the goals and rationale for culture transformation.

The translational phase utilized the PDSA methodology for practice improvement (the Deming cycle). Project champions were identified by the NICU leadership group and these champions formed subcommittees on each of the core measures for developmental care and executed tests of change for care practice improvements, which were then refined, revised, and incorporated into the unit's developmental care practice protocols and guidelines.

The evaluation phase began with a staff self-assessment survey evaluating the frequency with which staff provided developmentally supportive care as defined by the core measures. The frequency was set over a 5-point Likert-type scale ranging from *never* to *always*. The initial assessment was obtained prior to the education phase and follow-up assessments were obtained at 1 and 2 years posteducation session. Figure 11.1 demonstrates the trend in staff perceptions of the frequency with which the desired evidence-based best practices were provided across each core

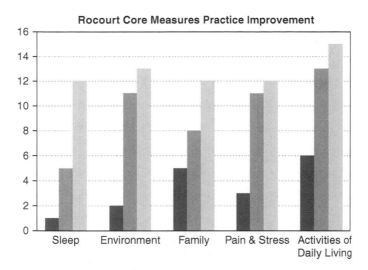

Figure 11.1 *Staff self-assessment of frequency with which developmental care practices aligned with the core measure metrics.*

Reprinted with permission from Maton and Francoise (2011).

measure category. Observations of clinical practice and chart audit confirmed these perceptions.

To evaluate whether or not the integration of the core measures into the culture of care would impact short-term and long-term outcomes, the team at the Rocourt NICU conducted an observational cohort study of infants with a gestational age of less than 32 weeks. The demographics of the benchmark and study cohorts were extracted 18 months prior to the education intervention; 18 months following the education intervention; and an additional period of 36 months following the education intervention referred to as Study Group 2. (Please see Table 11.1 for details regarding the cohort characteristics.)

Figure 11.2 highlights a statistically significant decrease in the incidence of intracranial hemorrhage Grades 1 and 2 in infants receiving care during the study periods; there is also a slight trend toward a decrease in the incidence of Grades 3 and 4 intracranial hemorrhages as well as periventricular leukomalacia. These findings warrant replication to confirm this trend, but are promising.

The data in Figure 11.3 present a very surprising effect of the cultural transformation—the statistically significant decrease in the incidence of gastroesophageal reflux. Diagnostic criteria remained the same across all

Table 11.1 *Patient Population Demographics*

	Before	Period 1	Period 2
Total	106	130	117
Male sex (%)	54 (50.9)	81 (62.3)	69 (58.9)
<26	4	11	17
26– <28	23	22	18
28– <32	79	97	82
Mean GA (SD)	28.9 (1.9)	28.7 (1.9)	28.9 (2.2)
Mean BW (SD)	1,226 (333)	1,331 (377)	1,250 (355)
Mean 5′ Apgar	7.9	7.9	8.1

Reprinted with permission from Maton and Francoise (2011).

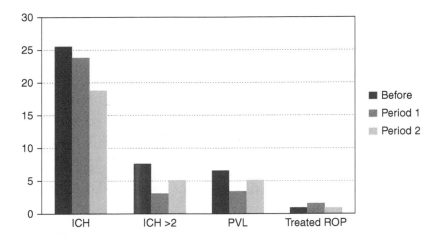

Figure 11.2 *Neurological outcomes (%).*

ICH, intracranial hemorrhage; PVL, periventricular leukomalacia; ROP, retinopathy of prematurity.
Reprinted with permission from Maton and Francoise (2011).

three periods and yet there is a greater than 50% reduction in the diagnosis of reflux.

Gastroesophageal reflux is a very common comorbidity observed in the hospitalized premature and critically ill infant. Pathogenic

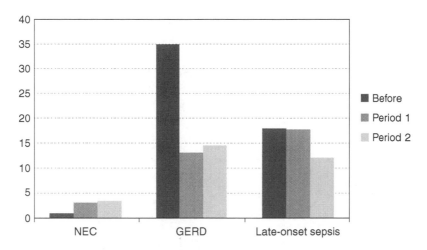

Figure 11.3 *Other outcomes (%).*

GERD, gastroesophageal reflux disease; NEC, necrotizing enterocolitis. Reprinted with permission from Maton and Francoise (2011).

mechanisms seem to be related to immaturity and also complicated by severity of illness; include transient relaxation of the lower esophageal sphincter, gastric emptying challenges, and esophageal motility; and are often exacerbated by respiratory disorders. Most premature/critically ill infants outgrow this condition by 1 year of age. Treatment options provided during NICU hospitalization, such as positioning strategies and pharmacological interventions, are not supported in the literature consistently and reliably. As such, the diagnosis of reflux can be frustrating and perplexing to NICU clinicians and infants. A greater than 50% decrease in the diagnosis of reflux suggests alternative pathogenic mechanisms that may be more responsive to treatment.

Konturek, Brzozowski, and Konturek (2011) indicate that gastroesophageal reflux represents one of the most important manifestations of stress exposure to the gastrointestinal (GI) tract. Activation of the hypothalamic–pituitary–adrenal (HPA) axis, or initiation of the fight or flight response, causes decreased perfusion to the GI tract and also changes lower esophageal sphincter tone. Through understanding hospitalization in the NICU as a developmental trauma and life stressor for the premature and critically ill infants, one can easily understand the link between stress and reflux. In addition, unmanaged or undermanaged pain as a stressor can compound the infant's vulnerability to gastroesophageal reflux. These findings do warrant replication but certainly do present a viable, noninvasive treatment strategy for the management of symptomatic reflux in the NICU.

With regard to length of hospital stay, the data suggest a trend toward a shorter length of stay, particularly in infants with a gestational age more than 26 weeks; average daily weight gain improved as well (Table 11.2).

Looking at the 2-year follow-up data (Table 11.3), it is interesting to note that a higher percentage of infants were available for evaluation and more of these infants from the study period were assessed as neurodevelopmentally normal (using BAPM criteria) than the baseline group (Figures 11.4 and 11.5).

Feeding problems did not seem to be impacted by the care practice changes (although this was not a focus of practice change during the study period); however, there were fewer children with respiratory disorders at 2 years, and this could be attributed to an increase in the use of surfactant during the project phase (Figure 11.6).

Table 11.2 *Length of Stay and Weight Gain*

	Before (106)	After (130)	After 2 (117)
Length of stay Mean ± SD	63.9 ± 17.7	61.5 ±20.8	63.7 ± 24.8
Length of stay Mean ± SD (>26 weeks)	63.4 ± 17.5	58.2 ±16.5	57.4 ± 17.6
Weight gain (g/day)	20.5	20.8	21.8

Reprinted with permission from Maton and Francoise (2011).

Table 11.3 *Rocourt 2-Year Follow-Up Cohort*

	Before (106)	After (130)
Discharged	91	120
Post neonatal death	1	0
Followed-up at 2 years	65 (71%)	102 (85%)

Reprinted with permission from Maton and Francoise (2011).

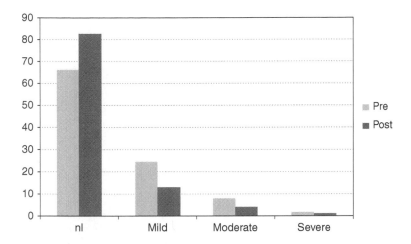

Figure 11.4 *Rocourt neurodisability at 2 years (%) per BAPM.*

Pre = outcomes of infants cared for in NICU before the unit adopted and integrated core measure practices; Post = outcomes of infants cared for in NICU after integration of evidence-based core measures for age-appropriate care practices. Reprinted with permission from Maton and Francoise (2011).

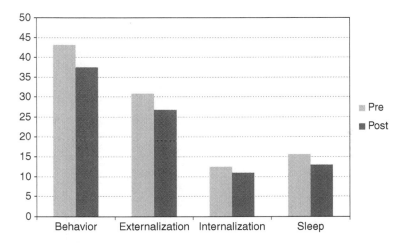

Figure 11.5 *Rocourt psychoemotional outcomes (%).*

Pre = outcomes of infants cared for in NICU before the unit adopted and integrated core measure practices; Post = outcomes of infants cared for in NICU after integration of evidence-based core measures for age-appropriate care practices. Reprinted with permission from Maton and Francoise (2011).

Parental confidence and competence are crucial elements to successful parenting. Having an infant who requires NICU hospitalization is a traumatic life event for parents, leading to feelings of helplessness and high stress levels that interfere with a couple's relationship, and also negatively

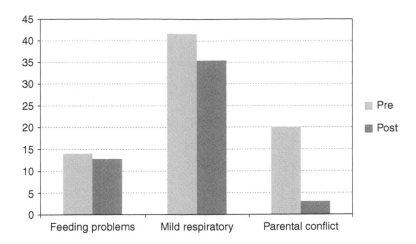

Figure 11.6 *Rocourt 2-year follow-up outcomes (%).*

Pre = outcomes of infants cared for in NICU before the unit adopted and integrated core measure practices; Post = outcomes of infants cared for in NICU after integration of evidence-based core measures for age-appropriate care practices. Reprinted with permission from Maton and Francoise (2011).

impacting the parent–infant interaction trajectory (Melnyk et al., 2006). The cultural transformation that occurred at the Rocourt NICU may have played a role in the 80% decrease in self-reported parental conflict in the study group. Family-centered care (FCC) is an integral component to the core measures; the family's role in caring and parenting during the hospitalization is reflected across each core measure set (Figure 11.6).

Additional Projects

Hooftman (2012), in an unpublished master's thesis, presents her work looking at reducing sound levels in a Level-III NICU following an education intervention, evaluating whether this reduction in noise levels impacts the infants' level of comfort (determined by Neonatal Pain, Agitation, and Sedation Scale [NPASS] scores), and also assessing whether this practice change affects the nurses' workload. The decision to employ the core measures was determined by a need to create standardization of practice, and the implementation methodology to create change associated with the core measures engaged *all* clinical staff.

Hooftman reports that through clearly defined metrics for success and engaging all disciplines in the practice change initiative, the department was able to reduce the sound levels in the NICU from 55 dB to

53 dB (p <.001). In observations during the baseline data collection, 11% of infants exhibited stress cues, compared to 9% in the postintervention group (p <.001). NPASS averaged 0.3 points lower in the postintervention group. In addition, staff respondents indicated that their workload decreased by 10% (p = .025). Job satisfaction was virtually unchanged (p = .133).

Backus and Roday (2011) presented their NICU journeys to improve their delivery of FCC practices. Using the core measures as their evidence-based best-practice standards, framed by the UDC model, the team aimed to increase the frequency of skin-to-skin contact, including kangaroo care and breast-feeding in their Level-III NICU. The selection of this approach to practice change was made based on the model's design to develop sustainability in cultural and practice changes that empowered and engaged staff.

Utilizing the PDSA model for improvement after staff education, the team was able to increase the frequency of skin-to-skin contact for all new admissions to the NICU, decrease the length of time from birth to the initial skin-to-skin experience, and increase breast-feeding rates. In addition, staff perceptions of the level of FCC provided tripled.

Lessons Learned

Change is difficult and requires vigilance, persistence, and accountability in order to transform a culture of care. All three of the referenced projects shared the challenges associated with changing behavior and sustaining behavioral change. Accountability is key to sustaining change, and this must happen on the frontline, peer-to-peer, role modeling the expected best practices.

Respectfully reminding colleagues about the selected practice change goals reinforces performance expectations and supports success in practice transformation. We all need reminders and we all need support.

Standardizing care strategies using evidence-based best practices across key human caring domains can streamline workflow and dramatically impact clinical outcomes across physiologic and psychoemotional indicators.

CHAPTER 12: *Implications for Best Practice in the NICU*

*I*n a health care environment driven by quality and safety, the implications for best practice become paramount. Providing evidence-based best practice in the neonatal intensive care unit (NICU) ensures that care delivery meets the highest standards.

Best practices in the NICU not only include diagnosis and disease management practices but also must incorporate best practices in age-appropriate care and prevention strategies. Understanding that a significant amount of disease-independent lifelong morbidity begins in the NICU, clinicians are charged with managing the precursors to these neonatal complications. Evidence-based preventative strategies begin with the adoption of the core measures for age-appropriate care.

STANDARDIZATION OF QUALITY CARING IN THE NICU

Standardizing quality caring actions, attitudes, and behaviors in the NICU is, to say the least, challenging in the high-tech, high-touch world of neonatology. Unlike changing a disease management protocol or a procedural intervention, quality caring actions, attitudes, and behaviors are mediated by human factors—empathy, compassion, and an acknowledgment of our shared humanity with others.

When these human components of caring are tangibly demonstrated consistently and reliably, a trusting milieu is created. This is a neonatal requisite for optimal psychoemotional and psychosocial development. Creating consistency in the experience of care reduces the stress associated with hospitalization and impacts short-term and long-term physiological and psychological outcomes for the fragile individuals served in the NICU.

> *True ethical care needs to elevate the actual person with sickness to the pedestal of priority, not the health care system or the disease management process.* —Nolan

The Value of Standardized Quality Caring

> *Our nation's ability to successfully compete in a global economy will suffer until we find solutions that can improve the health of all Americans and advance quality and control costs. We can, and we must, do better than ranking 37th among nations in population health status while spending twice as much money per citizen on health care services than other countries. Value-based purchasing strategies represent the path forward.* —Andrew Webber, president and CEO, National Business Coalition on Health

Value-based purchasing (VBP) is designed to promote quality and value in the provision of health care services. This strategy focuses on a return on investment associated with health care spend. For the consumer, this model aims to mitigate and even eliminate preventable adverse outcomes associated with hospitalization. For the organization, there is a financial gain in reducing preventable adverse outcomes, which benefits both the organization and the patient and drives market share to those who deliver on high quality consistently and reliably.

Improving patient outcomes seems obvious; of course, we want the best outcomes for our patients, right? Unfortunately, our current system is not oriented toward improved patient outcomes and a complication-free approach to care delivery. Our system is driven by revenue, and until we are able to incentivize providers and organizations to focus on quality, we will fail the patient every time. We must consciously shift from a "sick care" paradigm to a patient-centered, prevention-oriented model.

Eappen et al. (2013) published results of a retrospective analysis of administrative data for inpatient surgical discharges during 2010 across 12 nonprofit hospitals in the southern United States. The results demonstrated that postsurgical complications sustained by individuals resulted in a financial gain for the hospitals concerned. These types of findings undermine quality improvement initiatives and quality patient care delivery.

Despite these systematic challenges, however, all is not lost, as nurses are perfectly positioned to improve patient outcomes and the patient's experience of care. The Institute of Medicine's (IOM's) 2010 report, *The Future of Nursing: Leading Change, Advancing Health*, recommends a reconceptualization of the role of nursing, including health coaching, prevention activities, and quality improvement (IOM, 2011; Reinhard & Hassmiller, 2012). This reconceptualization is a reorientation to the roots of nursing, the Nightingale legacy. "Let whoever is in charge keep this simple question in her head (not, how can I always do this right thing myself, but) how can I provide for this right thing to be always done?" (Florence Nightingale, 1860).

For the neonatal patient population, "doing the right thing always" will prevent adverse events and impact short-term and lifelong outcomes—this is the role of the neonatal nurse.

> *The ultimate goal of neonatal intensive care is to provide survival without impairment.*—Hack

Patient Experience of Care in the NICU

Despite advances in understanding the physiological integrity and developmental requisites of the neonatal patient, this vulnerable population continues to endure experiences that no other patient population would tolerate. Attributes of the experience of care include but are not limited to pain, stress, isolation, sleep deprivation, as well as excessive and inappropriate sensory stimulation.

Barker and Rutter (1995) quantified the number of invasive procedures to a cohort of 54 infants admitted to a NICU, with gestation ages ranging from 23 to 41 weeks (median age 33 weeks). The total number of invasive procedures recorded were 3,283, of which 56% were heel stick blood sampling, 26% were endotracheal suctioning, and 8% were IV insertions. The most immature individuals experienced the highest number of procedures, with 74% of the total performed on infants less than 31 weeks gestation, and none of these procedures were managed for pain and or stress.

Simons et al. (2003), in a prospective study of procedural pain and analgesia use in neonates, concluded that although clinicians estimated that most NICU procedures are painful, only one third of the infants received appropriate analgesic therapy.

Answering the question "Can adverse neonatal experiences alter brain development and subsequent behavior?" Anand and Scalzo (2000) present a neurobiological model of cellular mechanisms that are adversely impacted by neonatal experiences in the NICU. These experiences include excessive stimulation from perinatal/neonatal trauma-inducing neuronal excitotoxicity in multiple areas of the developing brain, as well as a lack of appropriate sensory stimulation to enhance normal developmental apoptosis.

These deviations in neonatal brain development provide insight into the pathogenic mechanisms of the long-term behavioral, cognitive, and psychological outcomes seen in adolescents and adults with a history of NICU hospitalization. Anand and Scalzo highlight the public health importance of the NICU experience of care. Prevention strategies aimed at eliminating or at least minimizing the trauma experience, effectively managing stress and pain, and promoting age-appropriate experiences for this vulnerable population cannot be overemphasized.

Smith et al. (2011), in a prospective cohort study of infants less than 34 weeks gestation, were able to document regional alterations in brain structure and function with exposure to stressors during NICU hospitalization. The stressors identified included not only painful invasive procedures but also care interactions that have been described as routine. The researchers used the Neonatal Infant Stressor Scale (Newnham, Inder, & Milgrom, 2009), which lists 36 procedures and interventions identified to contribute to infant stress in the NICU, ranging from diaper change to endotracheal intubation. These findings highlight the profound need to decrease and mitigate exposure to stressors in the NICU and ensure an age-appropriate experience of care for the premature and critically ill infant.

Additional challenges of the NICU patient experience of care include environmental influences (light, sound, smell, taste, tactile, vestibular, and proprioceptive experiences), sleep deprivation, and maternal separation. Standardizing an age-appropriate experience of care that is consistently and reliably delivered has the potential to not only improve the patient's outcomes but also streamline nursing workflow.

In the pilot project evaluating the impact of the core measures for age-appropriate care (described in Chapter 11), the team in Rocourt Belgium discovered that despite an increase in patient census during the study period and working with the same number of nursing full-time equivalencies (FTEs), the patient's length of stay decreased, in addition to the reported clinical improvements (Figure 12.1).

Transformation of the culture of care with clearly articulated practice expectations related to the patient's age-appropriate needs, supported by frontline accountability, engaged and empowered the Rocourt bedside

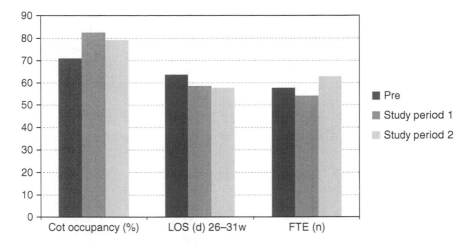

Figure 12.1 *Rocourt nurse workload.*

FTE, full-time equivalency; LOS, length of stay.

clinicians and streamlined workflow efficiencies, favorably impacting patient outcomes and staff satisfaction.

POPULATION HEALTH AND THE BURDEN OF DISEASE

Kindig and Stoddart (2003) proposed a definition of population health to be "the health outcomes of a group of individuals, including the distribution of such outcomes within the group" (p. 380). Embracing this definition, we can critically appraise the health outcomes associated with prematurity and neonatal critical illness within the context of the NICU experience, thus going beyond the primary admitting diagnosis to assess how the experience of hospitalization during a highly vulnerable life-stage influences the developmental health trajectory of this population.

Quantifying population health requires statistical analysis looking at mortality and morbidity across various disease categories. The statistical metric used by the World Health Organization (WHO) is the disability-adjusted life year (DALY), which calculates the impact of disease on lived years. DALY is equal to the sum of "years of life lost" (YLL) due to premature death and "years lost to disability" (YLD); so one DALY = one lost year of a healthy life. This calculation captures the burden of disease and aims to provide a deeper understanding of how health and quality of life are impacted across various disease entities.

Mathers and Loncar (2006) published projections of global mortality and burden of disease from 2002 to 2030. Perinatal conditions ranked first as the leading cause of DALY (burden of disease) in 2002 but are projected to fall to fifth place standing by 2030. This projection is based on assumptions about improvements in infant care over the next decade and a half. Interestingly, unipolar depressive disorder, ranked fourth in 2002 for burden of disease, is projected to be a leading cause of DALY in 2030 (second place). With more and more neonates surviving the NICU experience, and emerging research demonstrating the increased risk for psychopathological morbidity in this patient population, it stands to reason that NICU graduates may be contributing to the increasing global burden of mental illness.

Saigal and Doyle (2008) confirm that survival rates for younger individuals have improved significantly in the wake of technological advances and improved collaborations between obstetric and neonatal clinicians. However, given these improvements, there remains significant morbidity attached to NICU survivors. The authors suggest a focus on perinatal interventions aimed at reducing long-term morbidity by emphasizing preventative strategies to preserve neonatal brain development.

Protecting and preserving brain development in the neonatal patient population will go a long way in reducing the burden of disease globally associated with perinatal and mental health conditions. Using Anand and Scalzo's proposed cellular mechanisms for altered brain development and subsequent behavioral pathologies, we may answer Baxter, Patton, Scott, Degenhardt, and Whiteford's (2013) question "What are we missing?" related to the global epidemiology of mental disorders.

Long-Term Morbidities Associated With Prematurity and Neonatal Critical Illness

Disease-independent, long-term morbidity associated with NICU hospitalization includes physiologic and psychological sequelae. Research is now looking at epigenetic phenomena as a mediator of short-term and long-term complications. The developmental origins theory proposes that perinatal events and activation of the hypothalamic–pituitary–adrenal (HPA) axis provoke adaptive changes in psychoneuroendocrine processes that adversely impact adult health (Sullivan, Hawes, Winchester, & Miller, 2008). The sensitivity of the human epigenome to environmental influences is designed as an adaptive mechanism modifying metabolic and homeostatic systems; however, the immediate adaptations to early life insults are associated with later-life liabilities, including cardiovascular disease, diabetes, obesity, and neuropsychiatric disorders (Boekelheide et al., 2012).

Vanderbilt and Gleason (2010) present a very comprehensive review of mental health challenges of prematurity across the life span. Figure 12.2 highlights the key neurodevelopmental morbidities associated with prematurity. Summarizing the magnitude of neuropsychiatric and behavioral challenges that extend across the developmental continuum of the premature infant population, the authors alert child psychiatrists to the unique vulnerabilities and needs of this patient–family population.

Increased risk for neurodevelopmental disability or developmental delay is not only relegated to preterm infants. Marino et al. (2012) reviewed the available research addressing developmental disability and developmental delay in infants hospitalized for congenital heart disease and identified several categories that placed these infants at high risk for developmental disability. One noteworthy risk factor was prolonged hospitalization, defined as a postoperative length of stay of more than 2 weeks in the hospital. This risk factor suggests a relationship between developmental disability and the experience of care in the NICU.

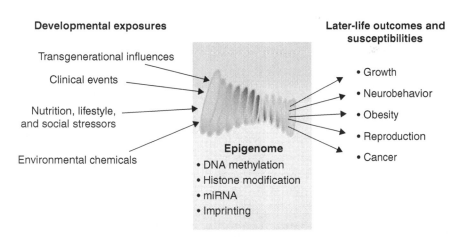

Figure 12.2 *Developmental exposures are focused through the lens of epigenetic mechanisms to influence later-life disease outcomes and susceptibilities.*

miRNA, micro-ribonucleic acid. Reprinted with permission from Boekelheide et al. (2012).

In addition to neurodevelopmental compromise, research reveals significant psychopathologic morbidity in the preterm patient population. Nosarti et al. (2012) employed an historical population-based cohort study and concluded that infants born prematurely had an increased risk of hospitalization across a range of psychiatric disorders (Exhibit 12.1).

Long-term morbidities associated with the NICU experience are not only linked to neurodevelopmental disability and psychological pathology, but also to cardiovascular and metabolic complications. Lewandowski et al. (2013) report that individuals born preterm exhibit left ventricular hypertrophy and alterations in systolic and diastolic function. In addition, the study cohort of young adults born premature were shorter in stature, weighed more, and had increased levels of low-density lipoprotein (LDL) cholesterol, triglyceride, glucose, and insulin levels on their metabolic panel when compared to the young adult term-born cohort.

As the first generation of NICU survivors from the surfactant era approach adulthood, evidence of prematurity as a risk factor for chronic kidney disease is becoming evident (Carmody & Charlton, 2013). The pathogenic mechanism for this emerging morbidity is linked to the developmental origins theory applied to nephrogenesis by Dr. Barry Brenner. Exposure to a variety of external stressors hinders ongoing kidney development and places these individuals at risk for adult ramifications of renal disease.

Understanding the precursors to neonatal complications and neonatal morbidity guides NICU clinicians in providing quality preventative

Exhibit 12.1 *Nosarti et al. (2012) Findings*

COMPARED WITH TERM BIRTHS
▦ Infants born at 32 to 36 weeks were:
● 1.6 × more likely to have nonaffective psychosis (schizophrenia)
● 1.3 × more likely to have depressive disorder
● 2.7 × more likely to have bipolar affective disorder
▦ Infants born at less than 32 weeks were:
● 2.5 × more likely to have nonaffective psychosis (schizophrenia)
● 2.9 × more likely to have depressive disorder
● 7.4 × more likely to have bipolar disorder

care to this highly vulnerable and susceptible population. Moore, Berger, and Wilson (2012) propose a model that frames the physiologic dysregulation associated with prematurity and critical illness, using the concepts of allostasis and adaptive–maladaptive physiologic response patterns.

Moore's model, although developed within the context of prematurity, can be applied to full-term critically ill neonates as well. Consistently and reliably mitigating and managing the stressors of the NICU experience of care is an effective, evidence-based intervention to reduce the burden of disease associated with the NICU patient population.

Quality of Life and Economic Costs of Prematurity and Neonatal Critical Illness

The quality of life and economic costs associated with these morbidities are difficult to measure. Meadow and Lantos (2009) present a comprehensive reflection on NICU care and share that the outcome data do not define cost-effectiveness. From an economic perspective, treatment interventions are considered cost-effective if they provide a quality-adjusted life year (QALY) for less than $50,000.00, and for infants born at even the lowest birth weight, each QALY cost was less than $10,000.00. Despite this apparent cost-effectiveness of immediate neonatal care, in light of the long-term sequelae and associated economic burden, more can be done to reduce the lifelong consequences. Zupancic (2007) presents a systematic review of costs associated with preterm birth that incorporates initial hospitalization costs with postdischarge expenses, educational expenses, as well as direct and indirect costs. The annual societal economic burden associated with preterm birth in the United States was at least $26.2 billion in 2005.

Hodek, von der Schulenburg, and Mittendorf (2011) captured financial as well as quality of life aspects associated with prematurity. Looking at financial burden of prematurity in a European context, studies confirm an inverse relationship between newborn care expenses and gestational age. Figure 12.3 represents the relationship between the average overall 2-year costs for surviving preterm infants (birth weight [BW], 1,000 g) compared with term births in Finland.

Health-related quality of life (HRQoL) is a subjective perception of health status on physical, emotional, and social functioning. For infants, parents or primary caregivers generally complete these quality of life assessments. These proxy versions generally indicate that the NICU

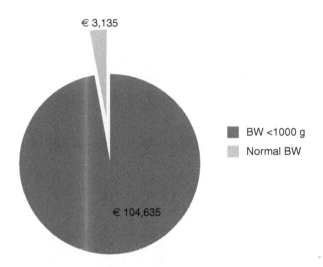

Figure 12.3 *Health care costs for the first 2 years of life.*

BW, birth weight.

survivor is significantly less healthy than his or her term counterparts. However, when these children or adolescents born preterm are interviewed they do not perceive their HRQoL much different from their peers.

Clements, Barfield, Ayadi, and Wilber (2007) attempt to capture economic and quality of life costs, analyzing the utilization of early intervention services in Massachusetts. Breaking down costs, based on service provider, shares insight into the global impact of prematurity on quality of life indicators.

Doyle and Anderson (2010) present a review of adult outcomes of extreme prematurity, and report across cardiovascular health, pulmonary function, neurosensory impairments, educational achievements, cognitive function, psychiatric disorders, quality of life, and functional outcomes. Overall, their findings confirm a higher rate of adverse health outcomes, which are linked to an additive economic burden for this patient population.

Mitigating Morbidities Through Trauma-Informed Age-Appropriate Care

Trauma-informed age-appropriate care places the person first with each and every care interaction and reflects the ideal patient experience of care for individuals hospitalized in the NICU. Grounded in the latest research on neurobiology and epigenetics, NICU clinicians hold the key to minimizing and mitigating the incidence of long-term morbidities associated with NICU hospitalization. However, creating an exceptional patient and family experience of care requires more than the actions of the bedside clinician.

The Institute for Healthcare Improvement outlines primary drivers necessary to achieve an exceptional patient experience of care.

▪ **Leadership**: Governance and executive leaders demonstrate that everything in the culture is focused on patient- and family-centered care practiced everywhere in the hospital—at the individual patient level, at the microsystem level, and across the organization, including governance.
▪ **Hearts and Minds**: The hearts and minds of staff and providers are fully engaged through respectful partnerships with everyone in the organization and in a commitment to the shared values of patient- and family-centered care.
▪ **Respectful Partnership**: Every care interaction is anchored in a respectful partnership, anticipating and responding to patient and family needs (e.g., physical, emotional, informational, cultural, spiritual, and educational).
▪ **Reliable Care**: Hospital systems deliver reliable, quality care 24/7.
▪ **Evidence-Based Care**: The care team instills confidence by providing collaborative, evidence-based care (the core measures for age-appropriate care). (Balik, Conway, Zipperer, & Watson, 2011)

To measurably impact short-term and long-term outcomes, a systematic approach is necessary to organize, engage, and empower all stakeholders. It is not enough for a few clinicians to incorporate the principles and practices of trauma-informed age-appropriate care into their care delivery repertoire; the practice model must be embraced, adopted, and implemented by all clinicians who interface with the infant–family dyad as well as by all staff who interface with the NICU environment.

Quality of Life Impact and Economic Benefits for Trauma-Informed Age-Appropriate Care

As demonstrated in Chapter 11, quality of life enhancements, as well as cost savings, can be deduced from the outcome data. The current available evidence is sufficient to require this model to become the true standard of care across NICUs worldwide.

Trauma-informed age-appropriate care is compassionate, patient-centered care. Lown, Rosen, and Marttila (2011) reviewed the data evaluating the impact of compassionate care on clinical and economic outcomes. Compassionate care is defined by:

> *Relationships based on empathy, emotional support, and efforts to understand and relieve the patient's discomfort and suffering; effective communication within interactions, over time, and across settings; respect for and facilitation of patients' and families' participation in decisions and care; and contextualized knowledge of the patient as an individual within a network of relationships at home and in the community.*—Lown et al.

The Schwartz Center for Compassionate Healthcare compiled a national survey of patients and physicians regarding the importance of compassionate care during the medical encounter. The majority of the respondents indicated that compassionate care was "very important" to medical treatment, yet only 53% of patients and 57% of physicians indicated that health care systems provide compassionate care. When compassionate care is provided, there is documented improvement in medical outcomes and patient satisfaction.

How much research is necessary to inform and transform our current practice?
I think we are there!

> *Unless someone like you cares a whole awful lot, nothing is going to get better. It's not.*—Dr. Seuss

CHAPTER 13: *Call to Action—Summary*

Providing evidence-based, trauma-informed age-appropriate care is a global health imperative. The actions we take now to care for this fragile patient population and their families will impact their future and the future of our global society. The legacy of Florence Nightingale and the grounded caring science of Jean Watson frame nurses' work and emphasize the caring dimensions of this work as fundamental in managing the experience of illness for vulnerable individuals.

Caring actions, attitudes, and behaviors improve patient outcomes. Managing and mitigating pain and stress, protecting neonatal sleep, creating a healing environment, and supporting parent–infant relationships in the neonatal intensive care unit (NICU) are examples of caring actions, attitudes, and behaviors. These actions for caring are in essence preventative strategies that have been demonstrated to affect key morbidities associated with NICU hospitalization (Gibbins, Coughlin, & Hoath, 2010; Maton et al., 2010; Maton & Francoise, 2011; Melnyk et al., 2006; Montirosso et al., 2012).

As outlined in the previous chapters, the deleterious effects of stress and trauma on the developing human are effectively managed through the consistently reliable delivery of trauma-informed age-appropriate care in the NICU.

By constantly seeking new ways to improve the care that we provide to patients, we can achieve positive change. *Everything matters.* The clinician's approach to the bedside, the introduction to the patient for a care interaction, the preparation to reduce stress and distress are just some of the opportunities to provide quality caring. Every care interaction makes

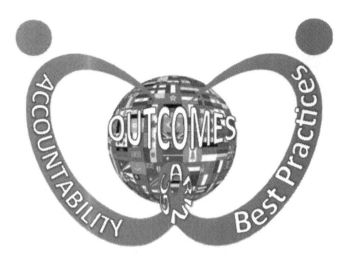

Figure 13.1 *Cultural transformation and quantum caring.*

an impression. Making the best impression every time requires a cultural transformation aimed at consistently providing quality caring through evidence-based best practices—trauma-informed age-appropriate care (Figure 13.1).

The concept of trauma-informed age-appropriate care provides clinicians with an understanding of the physiological, neurobiological, and psychoemotional challenges of the NICU experience for the premature and critically ill, hospitalized infant–family dyad and presents evidence-based strategies to confront these challenges. Implementation must be a quality priority for all stakeholders: individual clinicians, health care organizations, and government agencies.

Trauma-informed age-appropriate care aligns with the Institute of Medicine's (IOM) six aims for health care improvement:

Safety—"Patients should not be harmed by the care that is intended to help them" (IOM, 2001). Trauma-informed age-appropriate care is grounded in the concept of First Do No Harm.

Timely—Delays in providing appropriate care can impact patient safety. The provision of trauma-informed age-appropriate care should begin on admission, as delays expose the infant to unnecessary stress and trauma.

Effective—"Care that is based on the use of systematically acquired evidence to determine whether an intervention produces better outcomes than alternatives—including the alternative of doing nothing" (IOM, 2001). The content of this book provides the reader with the body of evidence to support the efficacy of trauma-informed age-appropriate care.

Efficient—As demonstrated in the Rocourt Belgium data, by standardizing evidence-based, age-appropriate care strategies, nursing workflow efficiencies and clinical outcomes were improved (Maton & Francoise, 2011).

Equitable—"The purpose of the health system is to continually reduce the burden of illness, injury, and disability, and to improve the health and functioning of the people of the United States" (IOM, 2001). Although written with regard to the United States, this purpose extends to all people across the globe. This statement highlights the need for standards and accountability for best practice with each and every patient encounter.

Patient centered—As defined by the Picker Institute, patient-centered care includes respect for the patient as an individual, coordination and integration of care, communication and education, physical comfort, emotional support, and family involvement. These tenets are reflected in the core measure for family-centered care.

In advancing the quality of service to the fragile individuals cared for in the NICU, we must commit to a prevention orientation to the patient experience of care, acknowledging the unique developmental vulnerabilities of this very special population.

> Touch a life…impact a lifetime. (Children's Healthcare of Atlanta, Egleston, and Scottish Rite Quantum Caring Teams, 2013)

Final examination for continuing nursing education credits can be accessed at the Quality Caring Institute Moodle Site. Go to moodle.caringessentials.org and select the course titled "Transformative Nursing in the NICU."

References

Aita, M., & Snider, L. (2003). The art of developmental care in the NICU: A concept analysis. *Journal of Advanced Nursing, 41*(3), 223–232.

Allen, K. A. (2012). Promoting and protecting infant sleep. *Advances in Neonatal Care, 12*(5), 288–291.

Allen, M., & Williams, G. (2011). Consciousness, plasticity, and connectomics: The role of intersubjectivity in human cognition. *Frontiers in Psychology, 2,* 20.

Allen, M. C., & Capute, A. J. (1990). Tone and reflex development before term. *Pediatrics, 85*(3, Pt. 2), 393–399.

Als, H. (1982). Towards a synactive theory of development: Promise for the assessment of infant individuality. *Infant Mental Health Journal, 3,* 229–243.

Als, H., Duffy, F. H., McAnulty, G. B., Rivkin, M. J., Vajapeyam, S., Mulkern, R. V., . . . Eichenwald, E. C. (2004). Early experience alters brain function and structure. *Pediatrics, 113*(4), 846–857.

Als, H., & Gilkerson, L. (1997). The role of relationship-based developmentally supportive newborn intensive care in strengthening outcome of preterm infants. *Seminars in Perinatology, 21*(3), 178–189.

American Academy of Pediatrics (AAP), Committee on Fetus and Newborn and Section on Surgery, Section on Anesthesiology and Pain Medicine, Canadian Paediatrics Society and Fetus and Newborn Committee. (2006). Prevention and management of pain in the neonate: An update. *Pediatrics, 118,* 2231–2241.

American Academy of Pediatrics: Committee on Environmental Health. (1997). Noise: A hazard for the fetus and newborn. *Pediatrics, 100*(4), 724–727.

American Nurses Association. (2010). *Code of ethics for nurses with interpretive statements.* Silver Spring, MD: nursingworld.org.

Anand, K. J., & Scalzo, F. M. (2000). Can adverse neonatal experiences alter brain development and subsequent behavior? *Biology of the Neonate, 77*(2), 69–82.

Ancora, G., Maranella, E., Aceti, A., Pierantoni, L., Grandi, S., Corvaglia, L., & Faldella, G. (2010). Effect of posture on brain hemodynamics in preterm newborns not mechanically ventilated. *Neonatology, 97*(3), 212–217.

Arduini, D., Rizzo, G., Giorlandino, C., Valensise, H., Dell'Acqua, S., & Romanini, C. (1986). The development of fetal behavioural states: A longitudinal study. *Prenatal Diagnosis, 6*(2), 117–124.

Association of Women's Health, Obstetric and Neonatal Nurses. (2007). *AWHONN Neonatal Skin Condition Score Tool.* Washington, DC: Author.

Aucott, S., Donohue, P. K., Atkins, E., & Allen, M. C. (2002). Neurodevelopmental care in the NICU. *Mental Retardation and Developmental Disabilities Research Reviews, 8*(4), 298–308.

Axelin, A., Salanterä, S., & Lehtonen, L. (2006). 'Facilitated tucking by parents' in pain management of preterm infants: A randomized crossover trial. *Early Human Development, 82*(4), 241–247.

Azevedo, F. A., Carvalho, L. R., Grinberg, L. T., Farfel, J. M., Ferretti, R. E., Leite, R. E., . . . Herculano-Houzel, S. (2009). Equal numbers of neuronal and nonneuronal cells make the human brain an isometrically scaled-up primate brain. *The Journal of Comparative Neurology, 513*(5), 532–541.

Backus, A., & Roday, L. (2011, January). *Changing culture. Changing practice.* Poster presented at the 24th Annual Gravens Conference on the Physical and Developmental Environment of the High Risk Infant, Clearwater Beach, FL.

Bahman Bijari, B., Iranmanesh, S., Eshghi, F., & Baneshi, M. R. (2012). Gentle human touch and Yakson: The effect on preterm's behavioral reactions. *ISRN Nursing, 2012,* 750363.

Balik, B., Conway, J., Zipperer, L., & Watson, J. (2011). *Achieving an exceptional patient and family experience of inpatient hospital care.* IHI Innovation Series white paper. Cambridge, MA: Institute for Healthcare Improvement.

Ballabh, P. (2010). Intraventricular hemorrhage in premature infants: Mechanism of disease. *Pediatric Research, 67*(1), 1–8.

Ballantyne, M., Benzies, K. M., & Trute, B. (2013). Depressive symptoms among immigrant and Canadian born mothers of preterm infants at neonatal intensive care discharge: A cross sectional study. *BMC Pregnancy & Childbirth, 13*(Suppl. 1), s11. Retrieved from http://www.ncbi.nlm.nih.gov/pmc/articles/PMC3561187

Barker, D. P., & Rutter, N. (1995). Exposure to invasive procedures in neonatal intensive care unit admissions. *Archives of Disease in Childhood, 72*(1), F47–F48.

Barlow, S. M. (2009). Oral and respiratory control for preterm feeding. *Current Opinion in Otolaryngology & Head and Neck Surgery, 17*(3), 179–186.

Bartocci, M., Bergqvist, L. L., Lagercrantz, H., & Anand, K. J. (2006). Pain activates cortical areas in the preterm newborn brain. *Pain, 122*(1–2), 109–117.

Bastiaansen, J. A., Thioux, M., & Keysers, C. (2009). Evidence for mirror systems in emotions. *Philosophical Transactions of the Royal Society of London. Series B, Biological Sciences, 364*(1528), 2391–2404.

Baxter, A. J., Patton, G., Scott, K. M., Degenhardt, L., & Whiteford, H. A. (2013). Global epidemiology of mental disorders: What are we missing? *PLoS One, 8*(6), e65514.

Beck, C. T. (2003). Recognizing and screening for postpartum depression in mothers of NICU infants. *Advances in Neonatal Care, 3*(1), 37–46.

Beggs, S., Currie, G., Salter, M. W., Fitzgerald, M., & Walker, S. M. (2012). Priming of adult pain responses by neonatal pain experience: Maintenance by central neuroimmune activity. *Brain, 135*(Pt. 2), 404–417.

Begum, E. A., Bonno, M., Ohtani, N., Yamashita, S., Tanaka, S., Yamamoto, H., ... Komada, Y. (2008). Cerebral oxygenation responses during kangaroo care in low birth weight infants. *BMC Pediatrics, 8*, 51. Retrieved from http://www.ncbi.nlm.nih.gov/pmc/articles/PMC2585079

Bellieni, C. V. (2012). Pain assessment in human fetus and infants. *The AAPS Journal, 14*(3), 456–461.

Benoit, D. (2004). Infant-parent attachment: Definition, types, antecedents, measurement and outcome. *Paediatrics & Child Health, 9*(8), 541–545.

Besedovsky, L., Lange, T., & Born, J. (2012). Sleep and immune function. *Pflügers Archiv: European Journal of Physiology, 463*(1), 121–137.

Bhutta, A. T., & Anand, K. J. (2002). Vulnerability of the developing brain. Neuronal mechanisms. *Clinics in Perinatology, 29*(3), 357–372.

Bicking, C., & Moore, G. A. (2012). Maternal perinatal depression in the neonatal intensive care unit: The role of the neonatal nurse. *Neonatal Network, 31*(5), 295–304.

Blomqvist, Y. T., Frölund, L., Rubertsson, C., & Nyqvist, K. H. (2013). Provision of Kangaroo Mother Care: Supportive factors and barriers perceived by parents. *Scandinavian Journal of Caring Sciences, 27*(2), 345–353.

Blume-Peytavi, U., Hauser, M., Stamatas, G. N., Pathirana, D., & Garcia Bartels, N. (2012). Skin care practices for newborns and infants: Review of the clinical evidence for best practices. *Pediatric Dermatology, 29*(1), 1–14.

Boekelheide, K., Blumberg, B., Chapin, R. E., Cote, I., Graziano, J. H., Janesick, A., ... Rogers, J. M. (2012). Predicting later-life outcomes of early-life exposures. *Environmental Health Perspectives, 120*(10), 1353–1361.

Bouza, H. (2009). The impact of pain in the immature brain. *Journal of Maternal-Fetal & Neonatal Medicine, 22*(9), 722–732.

Bowlby, J. (1969). *Attachment and loss: Volume 1. Attachment*. London, UK: Hogarth Press.

Brame, A. L., & Singer, M. (2010). Stressing the obvious? An allostatic look at critical illness. *Critical Care Medicine, 38*(10, Suppl.), S600–S607.

Brennan, T. A., Leape, L. L., Laird, N. M., Hebert, L., Localio, A. R., Lawthers, A. G., ... Hiatt, H. H. (1991). Incidence of adverse events and negligence in hospitalized patients. Results of the Harvard Medical Practice Study I. *The New England Journal of Medicine, 324*(6), 370–376.

Bretherton, I. (1992). The origins of attachment theory: John Bowlby and Mary Ainsworth. *Developmental Psychology, 28*, 759–775.

Brett, J., Staniszewska, S., Newburn, M., Jones, N., & Taylor, L. (2011). A systematic mapping review of effective interventions for communicating with, supporting and providing information to parents of preterm infants. *BMJ Open, 1*(1), e000023.

Brown, G. (2009). NICU noise and the preterm infant. *Neonatal Network, 28*(3), 165–173.

Brummelte, S., Grunau, R. E., Chau, V., Poskitt, K. J., Brant, R., Vinall, J., . . . Miller, S. P. (2012). Procedural pain and brain development in premature newborns. *Annals of Neurology, 71*(3), 385–396.

Buckley, T. M., & Schatzberg, A. F. (2005). On the interactions of the hypothalamic-pituitary-adrenal (HPA) axis and sleep: Normal HPA axis activity and circadian rhythm, exemplary sleep disorders. *The Journal of Clinical Endocrinology and Metabolism, 90*(5), 3106–3114.

Buettner-Schmidt, K., & Lobo, M. L. (2012). Social justice: A concept analysis. *Journal of Advanced Nursing, 68*(4), 948–958.

Byers, J. F. (2003). Components of developmental care and the evidence for their use in the NICU. *The American Journal of Maternal Child Nursing, 28*(3), 174–180; quiz 181.

Byrd, P. J., Gonzales, I., & Parsons, V. (2009). Exploring barriers to pain management in newborn intensive care units: A pilot survey of NICU nurses. *Advances in Neonatal Care, 9*(6), 299–306.

Bystrova, K., Ivanova, V., Edhborg, M., Matthiesen, A. S., Ransjö-Arvidson, A. B., Mukhamedrakhimov, R., . . . Widström, A. M. (2009). Early contact versus separation: Effects on mother-infant interaction one year later. *Birth* (Berkeley, Calif.), *36*(2), 97–109.

Calkins, S. D., & Hill, A. (2007). Caregiver influences on emerging emotion regulations: Biological and environmental transactions in early development. In J. J Gross (Ed.), *Handbook of emotion regulation* (pp. 229–248). New York, NY: Guilford Press.

Campbell-Yeo, M., Fernandes, A., & Johnston, C. (2011). Procedural pain management for neonates using nonpharmacological strategies: Part 2: Mother-driven interventions. *Advances in Neonatal Care, 11*(5), 312–318, quiz p. 319.

Canadian Pediatrics Society. (2000). Prevention and management of pain and stress in the neonate. *Paediatrics & Child Health, 5*(1), 31–38.

Carbajal, R., Eble, B., & Anand, K. J. (2007). Premedication for tracheal intubation in neonates: Confusion or controversy? *Seminars in Perinatology, 31*(5), 309–317.

Carbajal, R., Rousset, A., Danan, C., Coquery, S., Nolent, P., Ducrocq, S., . . . Bréart, G. (2008). Epidemiology and treatment of painful procedures in neonates in intensive care units. *The Journal of the American Medical Association, 300*(1), 60–70.

Carceller-Blanchard, A., Cousineau, J., & Delvin, E. E. (2009). Point of care testing: Transcutaneous bilirubinometry in neonates. *Clinical Biochemistry, 42*(3), 143–149.

Carmody, J. B., & Charlton, J. R. (2013). Short-term gestation, long-term risk: Prematurity and chronic kidney disease. *Pediatrics, 131*(6), 1168–1179.

Carter, C. S. (2003). Developmental consequences of oxytocin. *Physiology & Behavior, 79*(3), 383–397.

Carter, M. A. (2009). Trust, power, and vulnerability: A discourse on helping in nursing. *The Nursing Clinics of North America, 44*(4), 393–405.

Caskey, M., Stephens, B., Tucker, R., & Vohr, B. (2011). Importance of parent talk on the development of preterm infant vocalizations. *Pediatrics, 128*(5), 910–916.

Castiello, U., Becchio, C., Zoia, S., Nelini, C., Sartori, L., Blason, L.,...Gallese, V. (2010). Wired to be social: The ontogeny of human interaction. *PLoS One, 5*(10), e13199.

Chock, V. Y., Ramamoorthy, C., & Van Meurs, K. P. (2012). Cerebral autoregulation in neonates with a hemodynamically significant patent ductus arteriosus. *The Journal of Pediatrics, 160*(6), 936–942.

Choiniere, D. B. (2010). The effects of hospital noise. *Nursing Administration Quarterly, 34*(4), 327–333.

Chu, A. T., & Lieberman, A. F. (2010). Clinical implications of traumatic stress from birth to age five. *Annual Review of Clinical Psychology, 6*, 469–494.

Cignacco, E. L., Sellam, G., Stoffel, L., Gerull, R., Nelle, M., Anand, K. J., & Engberg, S. (2012). Oral sucrose and "facilitated tucking" for repeated pain relief in preterms: A randomized controlled trial. *Pediatrics, 129*(2), 299–308.

Cisneros, K. A., Coker, K., DuBuisson, A. B., Swett, B., & Edwards, W. H. (2003). Implementing potentially better practices for improving family-centered care in neonatal intensive care units: Successes and challenges. *Pediatrics, 111*(4), e450–e460.

Clarac, F., Vinay, L., Cazalets, J. R., Fady, J. C., & Jamon, M. (1998). Role of gravity in the development of posture and locomotion in the neonatal rat. *Brain Research. Brain Research Reviews, 28*(1–2), 35–43.

Clements, K. M., Barfield, W. D., Ayadi, M. F., & Wilber, N. (2007). Preterm birth-associated cost of early intervention services: An analysis by gestational age. *Pediatrics, 119*(4), e866–e874.

Cole, P. M., Michel, M. K., & Teti, L. O. (1994). The development of emotion regulation and dysregulation: A clinical perspective. *Monographs of the Society for Research in Child Development, 59*(2–3), 73–100.

Collett, B. R., Aylward, E. H., Berg, J., Davidoff, C., Norden, J., Cunningham, M. L., & Speltz, M. L. (2012). Brain volume and shape in infants with deformational plagiocephaly. *Child's Nervous System, 28*(7), 1083–1090.

Comaru, T., & Miura, E. (2009). Postural support improves distress and pain during diaper change in preterm infants. *Journal of Perinatology, 29*(7), 504–507.

Committee on Psychosocial Aspects of Child and Family Health, Adoption, Dependent Care and Section on Development and Behavioral Pediatrics. (2012). Early childhood adversity, toxic stress, and the role of the pediatrician: Translating developmental science into lifelong health. *Pediatrics, 129*, e224–e231.

Cone, S., Pickler, R. H., Grap, M. J., McGrath, J., & Wiley, P. M. (2013). Endotracheal suctioning in preterm infants using four-handed versus routine care. *Journal of Obstetric, Gynecologic, and Neonatal Nursing, 42*(1), 92–104.

Corlett, J., & Twycross, A. (2006). Negotiation of parental roles within family-centred care: A review of the research. *Journal of Clinical Nursing, 15*(10), 1308–1316.

Coughlan, R. (2006). The socio-politics of technology and innovation: Problematizing the "caring" in healthcare? *Social Theory & Health, 4,* 334–352.

Coughlin, M. (2011). *Age-appropriate care of the premature and critically ill hospitalized infant: Guideline for practice.* Glenview, IL: National Association of Neonatal Nurses.

Coughlin, M., Gibbins, S., & Hoath, S. (2009). Core measures for developmentally supportive care in neonatal intensive care units: Theory, precedence and practice. *Journal of Advanced Nursing, 65*(10), 2239–2248.

Coughlin, M., Lohman, M. B., & Gibbins, S. (2010). Reliability and effectiveness of an infant positioning assessment tool to standardize developmentally supportive positioning practices in the neonatal intensive care unit. *Newborn and Infant Nursing Reviews, 10*(2), 104–106.

Cuesta, J. M., & Singer, M. (2012). The stress response and critical illness: A review. *Critical Care Medicine, 40*(12), 3283–3289.

Curley, M. A., Meyer, E. C., Scoppettuolo, L. A., McGann, E. A., Trainor, B. P., Rachwal, C. M., & Hickey, P. A. (2012). Parent presence during invasive procedures and resuscitation: Evaluating a clinical practice change. *American Journal of Respiratory and Critical Care Medicine, 186*(11), 1133–1139.

Curtin, L. (2010). Quantum nursing. *American Nurse Today, 5*(9), 71–72.

Davidge, S. T., Morton, J. S., & Rueda-Clausen, C. F. (2008). Oxygen and perinatal origins of adulthood diseases: Is oxidative stress the unifying element? *Hypertension, 52*(5), 808–810.

Davidson, R. J., & McEwen, B. S. (2012). Social influences on neuroplasticity: Stress and interventions to promote well-being. *Nature Neuroscience, 15*(5), 689–695.

Davydow, D. S., Katon, W. J., & Zatzick, D. F. (2009). Psychiatric morbidity and functional impairments in survivors of burns, traumatic injuries, and ICU stays for other critical illnesses: A review of the literature. *International Review of Psychiatry, 21*(6), 531–538.

Davydow, D. S., Richardson, L. P., Zatzick, D. F., & Katon, W. J. (2010). Psychiatric morbidity in pediatric critical illness survivors: A comprehensive review of the literature. *Archives of Pediatrics & Adolescent Medicine, 164*(4), 377–385.

Decety, J. (2010). The neurodevelopment of empathy in humans. *Developmental Neuroscience, 32*(4), 257–267.

DeFrino, D. T. (2009). A theory of the relational work of nurses. *Research and Theory for Nursing Practice, 23*(4), 294–311.

de Vries, J. I., & Fong, B. F. (2006). Normal fetal motility: An overview. *Ultrasound in Obstetrics & Gynecology, 27*(6), 701–711.

Dieter, J. N., Field, T., Hernandez-Reif, M., Emory, E. K., & Redzepi, M. (2003). Stable preterm infants gain more weight and sleep less after five days of massage therapy. *Journal of Pediatric Psychology, 28*(6), 403–411.

Dingeman, R. S., Mitchell, E. A., Meyer, E. C., & Curley, M. A. (2007). Parent presence during complex invasive procedures and cardiopulmonary resuscitation: A systematic review of the literature. *Pediatrics, 120*(4), 842–854.

Dionne, G., Touchette, E., Forget-Dubois, N., Petit, D., Tremblay, R. E., Montplaisir, J. Y., & Boivin, M. (2011). Associations between sleep-wake consolidation and language development in early childhood: A longitudinal twin study. *Sleep, 34*(8), 987–995.

Doheny, L., Hurwitz, S., Insoft, R., Ringer, S., & Lahav, A. (2012). Exposure to biological maternal sounds improves cardiorespiratory regulation in extremely preterm infants. *The Journal of Maternal-Fetal and Neonatal Medicine, 25*(9), 1591–1594.

Doheny, L., Morey, J. A., Ringer, S. A., & Lahav, A. (2012). Reduced frequency of apnea and bradycardia episodes caused by exposure to biological maternal sounds. *Pediatrics International, 54*(2), e1–e3.

Dougherty, D., & Luther, M. (2008). Birth to breast—a feeding care map for the NICU: Helping the extremely low birth weight infant navigate the course. *Neonatal Network, 27*(6), 371–377.

Douglas, A. J. (2010). Baby love? Oxytocin-dopamine interactions in mother-infant bonding. *Endocrinology, 151*(5), 1978–1980.

Doyle, L. W., & Anderson, P. J. (2010). Adult outcome of extremely preterm infants. *Pediatrics, 126*(2), 342–351.

Duffy, J. F., & Czeisler, C. A. (2009). Effect of light on human circadian physiology. *Sleep Medicine Clinics, 4*(2), 165–177.

Duffy, J. R. (2009). Caring for self. In J. R. Duffy, *Quality caring in nursing* (pp. 47–62). New York, NY: Springer Publishing Company.

Duhn, L. J., & Medves, J. M. (2004). A systematic integrative review of infant pain assessment tools. *Advances in Neonatal Care, 4*(3), 126–140.

Durackova, Z. (2010). Some insights into oxidative stress. *Physiological Research, 59*(4), 459–469.

Eappen, S., Lane, B. H., Rosenberg, B., Lipsitz, S. A., Sadoff, D., Matheson, D.,...Gawande, A. A. (2013). Relationship between occurrence of surgical complications and hospital finances. *The Journal of the American Medical Association, 309*(15), 1599–1606.

Ednick, M., Cohen, A. P., McPhail, G. L., Beebe, D., Simakajornboon, N., & Amin, R. S. (2009). A review of the effects of sleep during the first year of life on cognitive, psychomotor, and temperament development. *Sleep, 32*(11), 1449–1458.

Eggenberger, S. K., & Nelms, T. P. (2007). Being family: The family experience when an adult member is hospitalized with a critical illness. *Journal of Clinical Nursing, 16*(9), 1618–1628.

Eliakim, A., Nemet, D., Friedland, O., Dolfin, T., & Regev, R. H. (2002). Spontaneous activity in premature infants affects bone strength. *Journal of Perinatology, 22*(8), 650–652.

Engler, A. J., Ludington-Hoe, S. M., Cusson, R. M., Adams, R., Bahnsen, M., Brumbaugh, E.,...Williams, D. (2002). Kangaroo care: National survey of practice, knowledge, barriers, and perceptions. *The American Journal of Maternal Child Nursing, 27*(3), 146–153.

Esch, T., & Stefano, G. B. (2011). The neurobiological link between compassion and love. *Medical Science Monitor, 17*(3), RA65–RA75.

Espezel, H. J., & Canam, C. J. (2003). Parent-nurse interactions: Care of hospital-ized children. *Journal of Advanced Nursing, 44*(1), 34–41.

Favero, L., Pagliuca, L. M., & Lacerda, M. R. (2013). Transpersonal caring in nursing: An analysis grounded in a conceptual model. *Revista da Escola de Enfermagem, 47*(2), 489–494.

Feldman, R., Weller, A., Sirota, L., & Eidelman, A. I. (2002). Skin-to-skin contact (kangaroo care) promotes self-regulation in premature infants: Sleep-wake cyclicity, arousal modulation, and sustained exploration. *Developmental Psychology, 38*(2), 194–207.

Fernandes, A., Campbell-Yeo, M., & Johnston, C. C. (2011). Procedural pain man-agement for neonates using nonpharmacological strategies: Part 1: Sensorial interventions. *Advances in Neonatal Care, 11*(4), 235–241.

Ferrari, F., Bertoncelli, N., Gallo, C., Roversi, M. F., Guerra, M. P., Ranzi, A., & Hadders-Algra, M. (2007). Posture and movement in healthy preterm infants in supine position in and outside the nest. *Archives of Disease in Childhood, 92*(5), F386–F390.

Field, T., Diego, M., & Hernandez-Reif, M. (2010). Preterm infant massage ther-apy research: A review. *Infant Behavior & Development, 33*(2), 115–124.

Fitzgerald, M., & Walker, S. M. (2009). Infant pain management: A develop-mental neurobiological approach. *Nature Clinical Practice. Neurology, 5*(1), 35–50.

Flacking, R., Lehtonen, L., Thomson, G., Axelin, A., Ahlqvist, S., Moran, V. H.,...Dykes, F.; Separation and Closeness Experiences in the Neonatal Environment (SCENE) group. (2012). Closeness and separation in neonatal intensive care. *Acta Paediatrica, 101*(10), 1032–1037.

Fogel, A., de Koeyer, I., Bellagamba, F., & Bell, H. (2002). The dialogical self in the first two years of life: Embarking on a journey of discovery. *Theory & Psychology, 12*(2), 191–205.

Forcada-Guex, M., Pierrehumbert, B., Borghini, A., Moessinger, A., & Muller-Nix, C. (2006). Early dyadic patterns of mother-infant interactions and out-comes of prematurity at 18 months. *Pediatrics, 118*(1), e107–e114.

Franck, L. S., & Bruce, E. (2009). Putting pain assessment into practice: Why is it so painful? *Pain Research & Management, 14*(1), 13–20.

Franck, L. S., Oulton, K., & Bruce, E. (2012). Parental involvement in neonatal pain management: An empirical and conceptual update. *Journal of Nursing Scholarship, 44*(1), 45–54.

Franck, L. S., Oulton, K., Nderitu, S., Lim, M., Fang, S., & Kaiser, A. (2011). Parent involvement in pain management for NICU infants: A randomized con-trolled trial. *Pediatrics, 128*(3), 510–518.

Fryers, T., & Brugha, T. (2013). Childhood determinants of adult psychiatric dis-order. *Clinical Practice and Epidemiology in Mental Health, 9*, 1–50.

Fucile, S., McFarland, D. H., Gisel, E. G., & Lau, C. (2012). Oral and nonoral sensorimotor interventions facilitate suck-swallow-respiration functions and their coordination in preterm infants. *Early Human Development, 88*(6), 345–350.

Gallese, V. (2003). The manifold nature of interpersonal relations: The quest for a common mechanism. *Philosophical Transactions of the Royal Society of London. Series B, Biological Sciences, 358*(1431), 517–528.

Ganz, F. D. (2012). Sleep and immune function. *Critical Care Nurse, 32*(2), e19–e25.

Gelfer, P., Cameron, R., Masters, K., & Kennedy, K. A. (2013). Integrating "Back to Sleep" recommendations into neonatal ICU practice. *Pediatrics, 131*(4), e1264–e1270.

Gephart, S. M., & Cholette, M. (2012). P.U.R.E. Communication: A strategy to improve care-coordination for high risk birth. *Newborn and Infant Nursing Reviews, 12*(2), 109–114.

Gerber, R. J., Wilks, T., & Erdie-Lalena, C. (2010). Developmental milestones: Motor development. *Pediatrics in Review/American Academy of Pediatrics, 31*(7), 267–76; quiz 277.

Gertner, S., Greenbaum, C. W., Sadeh, A., Dolfin, Z., Sirota, L., & Ben-Nun, Y. (2002). Sleep-wake patterns in preterm infants and 6 month's home environment: Implications for early cognitive development. *Early Human Development, 68*(2), 93–102.

Gewolb, I. H., & Vice, F. L. (2006). Maturational changes in the rhythms, patterning, and coordination of respiration and swallow during feeding in preterm and term infants. *Developmental Medicine and Child Neurology, 48*(7), 589–594.

Gibbins, S., Coughlin, M., & Hoath, S. (2010). Quality indicators for developmental care: Using the universe of developmental care model as an exemplar for change. In C. Kenner & J. McGrath (Eds.), *Developmental care of newborns and infants: A guide for health professionals* (2nd ed., pp. 43–59). Glenview, IL: National Association of Neonatal Nurses.

Gibbins, S., Hoath, S. B., Coughlin, M., Gibbins, A., & Franck, L. (2008). The universe of developmental care: A new conceptual model for application in the neonatal intensive care unit. *Advances in Neonatal Care, 8*(3), 141–147.

Gilad, E., & Arnon, S. (2010). The role of live music and singing as a stress-reducing modality in the neonatal intensive care unit environment. *Music and Medicine, 2*(1), 18–22.

Gitto, E., Pellegrino, S., Manfrida, M., Aversa, S., Trimarchi, G., Barberi, I., & Reiter, R. J. (2012). Stress response and procedural pain in the preterm newborn: The role of pharmacological and non-pharmacological treatments. *European Journal of Pediatrics, 171*(6), 927–933.

Godkin, J. (2001). Healing presence. *Journal of Holistic Nursing, 19*(1), 5–21; quiz 22.

Goldfarb, W. (1945). Effects of psychological deprivation in infancy and subsequent adjustment. *American Journal of Psychiatry, 102*, 18–33.

Golec, L. (2009). The art of inconsistency: Evidence-based practice my way. *Journal of Perinatology, 29*(9), 600–602.

Gooding, J. S., Cooper, L. G., Blaine, A. I., Franck, L. S., Howse, J. L., & Berns, S. D. (2011). Family support and family-centered care in the neonatal intensive care unit: Origins, advances, impact. *Seminars in Perinatology, 35*(1), 20–28.

Gorovitz, S. (1994). Is caring a viable component of health care? *Health Care Analysis, 2*(2), 129–133.

Grasso, D. J., Ford, J. D., & Briggs-Gowan, M. J. (2013). Early life trauma exposure and stress sensitivity in young children. *Journal of Pediatric Psychology, 38*(1), 94–103.

Graven, S. N., & Browne, J. V. (2008a). Sensory development in the fetus, neonate and infant: Introduction and overview. *Newborn and Infant Nursing Reviews, 8*(4), 169–172.

Graven, S. N., & Browne, J. V. (2008b). Sleep and brain development: The critical role of sleep in fetal and early neonatal brain development. *Newborn and Infant Nursing Reviews, 8*(4), 173–179.

Grazel, R., Phalen, A. G., & Polomano, R. C. (2010). Implementation of the American Academy of Pediatrics recommendations to reduce sudden infant death syndrome risk in neonatal intensive care units: An evaluation of nursing knowledge and practice. *Advances in Neonatal Care, 10*(6), 332–342.

Greisen, G., Mirante, N., Haumont, D., Pierrat, V., Pallás-Alonso, C. R., Warren, I., . . . Cuttini, M.; ESF Network. (2009). Parents, siblings and grandparents in the Neonatal Intensive Care Unit. A survey of policies in eight European countries. *Acta Paediatrica, 98*(11), 1744–1750.

Grenier, I. R., Bigsby, R., Vergara, E. R., & Lester, B. M. (2003). Comparison of motor self-regulatory and stress behaviors of preterm infants across body positions. *The American Journal of Occupational Therapy, 57*(3), 289–297.

Grunau, R. (2002). Early pain in preterm infants. A model of long-term effects. *Clinics in Perinatology, 29*(3), 373–394, vii.

Grunau, R. E., Holsti, L., Haley, D. W., Oberlander, T., Weinberg, J., Solimano, A., . . . Yu, W. (2005). Neonatal procedural pain exposure predicts lower cortisol and behavioral reactivity in preterm infants in the NICU. *Pain, 113*(3), 293–300.

Grunau, R. E., Holsti, L., & Peters, J. W. (2006). Long-term consequences of pain in human neonates. *Seminars in Fetal & Neonatal Medicine, 11*(4), 268–275.

Grunau, R. E., Weinberg, J., & Whitfield, M. F. (2004). Neonatal procedural pain and preterm infant cortisol response to novelty at 8 months. *Pediatrics, 114*(1), e77–e84.

Guillaume, S., Michelin, N., Amrani, E., Benier, B., Durrmeyer, X., Lescure, S., . . . Caeymaex, L. (2013). Parents' expectations of staff in the early bonding process with their premature babies in the intensive care setting: A qualitative multicenter study with 60 parents. *BMC Pediatrics, 13*, 18.

Hack, M. (1999). Consideration of the use of health status, functional outcome, and quality-of-life to monitor neonatal intensive care practice. *Pediatrics, 103*(1, Suppl. E), 319–328.

Hack, M. (2009). Care of preterm infants in the neonatal intensive care unit. *Pediatrics, 123*(4), 1246–1247.

Harlow, H. F. (1958). The nature of love. *American Psychologist, 13*, 673–685.

Harlow, H. F., & Zimmermann, R. R. (1959). Affectional responses in the infant monkey. *Science, 130*, 421–432.

Harvey, M. E., & Pattison, H. M. (2012). Being there: A qualitative interview study with fathers present during the resuscitation of their baby at delivery. *Archives of Disease in Childhood, 97*(6), F439–F443.

Hebb, D. O. (1949). *The organization of behavior.* New York, NY: Wiley.

Heidenreich, P. A., Trogdon, J. G., Khavjou, O. A., Butler, J., Dracup, K., Ezekowitz, M. D., … Woo, Y. J.; American Heart Association Advocacy Coordinating Committee; Stroke Council; Council on Cardiovascular Radiology and Intervention; Council on Clinical Cardiology; Council on Epidemiology and Prevention; Council on Arteriosclerosis; Thrombosis and Vascular Biology; Council on Cardiopulmonary; Critical Care; Perioperative and Resuscitation; Council on Cardiovascular Nursing; Council on the Kidney in Cardiovascular Disease; Council on Cardiovascular Surgery and Anesthesia, and Interdisciplinary Council on Quality of Care and Outcomes Research. (2011). Forecasting the future of cardiovascular disease in the United States: A policy statement from the American Heart Association. *Circulation, 123*(8), 933–944.

Heinemann, A. B., Hellström-Westas, L., & Hedberg Nyqvist, K. (2013). Factors affecting parents' presence with their extremely preterm infants in a neonatal intensive care room. *Acta Paediatrica, 102*(7), 695–702.

Hendricks-Muñoz, K. D., & Prendergast, C. C. (2007). Barriers to provision of developmental care in the neonatal intensive care unit: Neonatal nursing perceptions. *American Journal of Perinatology, 24*(2), 71–77.

Hendricks-Muñoz, K. D., Li, Y., Kim, Y. S., Prendergast, C. C., Mayers, R., & Louie, M. (2013). Maternal and neonatal nurse perceived value of Kangaroo Mother Care and maternal care partnership in the neonatal intensive care unit. *American Journal of Perinatology, 30*(10), 875–880.

Heraghty, J. L., Hilliard, T. N., Henderson, A. J., & Fleming, P. J. (2008). The physiology of sleep in infants. *Archives of Disease in Childhood, 93*(11), 982–985.

Hoath, S. B., & Narendran, V. (2001). Development of the epidermal barrier. *NeoReviews, 2*(12), e269–e281.

Hodek, J.-M., von der Schulenburg, J.-M., & Mittendorf, T. (2011). Measuring economic consequences of preterm birth—methodological recommendations for the evaluation of personal burden on children and their caregivers. *Health Economics Review, 1*, 6. Retrieved from http://www.healtheconomicsreview.com/content/1/1/6

Hoffmann, A., & Spengler, D. (2012). The lasting legacy of social stress on the epigenome of the hypothalamic-pituitary-adrenal axis. *Epigenomics, 4*(4), 431–444.

Hogan, B. K. (2013). Caring as a scripted discourse versus caring as an expression of an authentic relationship between self and other. *Issues in Mental Health Nursing, 34*, 375–379.

Holditch-Davis, D., & Edwards, L. J. (1998). Modeling development of sleep-wake behaviors. II. Results of two cohorts of preterms. *Physiology & Behavior, 63*(3), 319–328.

Holditch-Davis, D., Scher, M., Schwartz, T., & Hudson-Barr, D. (2004). Sleeping and waking state development in preterm infants. *Early Human Development, 80*(1), 43–64.

Holsti, L., Grunau, R. E., & Shany, E. (2011). Assessing pain in preterm infants in the neonatal intensive care unit: Moving to a 'brain-oriented' approach. *Pain Management, 1*(2), 171–179.

Holsti, L., Grunau, R. E., Whifield, M. F., Oberlander, T. F., & Lindh, V. (2006). Behavioral responses to pain are heightened after clustered care in preterm infants born between 30 and 32 weeks gestational age. *The Clinical Journal of Pain, 22*(9), 757–764.

Hooftman, E. (2012). *Zorgt de implementatie van nieuwe richtlijnen op een NICU voor een reductie van het geluid en stress op de afdeling?* [Ensures the implementation of new guidelines in an NICU for a reduction of the noise and stress on the department?] (Unpublished master's thesis). University of Antwerp, Antwerp, Belgium.

Imeri, L., & Opp, M. R. (2009). How (and why) the immune system makes us sleep. *Nature Reviews Neuroscience, 10*(3), 199–210.

Institute of Medicine (IOM). (2001). *Crossing the quality chasm: A new health system for the 21st century.* New York, NY: The National Academies Press.

Institute of Medicine (IOM). (2011). *The future of nursing: Leading change, advancing health.* Washington, DC: The National Academies Press.

Jarrín, O. F. (2012). The integrality of situated caring in nursing and the environment. *ANS. Advances in Nursing Science, 35*(1), 14–24.

Jefferies, A. L.; Canadian Paediatric Society, Fetus and Newborn Committee. (2012). Kangaroo care for the preterm infant and family. *Paediatrics & Child Health, 17*(3), 141–146.

Jha, A. K., Orav, E. J., Li, Z., & Epstein, A. M. (2007). The inverse relationship between mortality rates and performance in the Hospital Quality Alliance measures. *Health Affairs, 26*(4), 1104–1110.

Johnson, B. H., Abraham, M. R., & Shelton, T. L. (2009). Patient- and family-centered care: Partnerships for quality and safety. *North Carolina Medical Journal, 70*(2), 125–130.

Johnson, D. E., & Gunner, M. R. (2011). Growth failure in institutionalized children. *Monographs of the Society for Research in Child Development, 76*(4), 92–126.

Johnston, C. C., Fernandes, A. M., & Campbell-Yeo, M. (2011). Pain in neonates is different. *Pain, 152*(3, Suppl.), S65–S73.

Johnstone, M. J. (2011). Nursing and justice as a basic human need. *Nursing Philosophy, 12*(1), 34–44.

The Joint Commission. (2008, July 9). Behaviors that undermine a culture of safety. *Sentinel Event Alert,* Issue 40, 1–3.

Jones, L., Woodhouse, D., & Rowe, J. (2007). Effective nurse parent communication: A study of parents' perceptions in the NICU environment. *Patient Education and Counseling, 69*(1–3), 206–212.

Jones, L. R. (2012). Oral feeding readiness in the neonatal intensive care unit. *Neonatal Network, 31*(3), 148–155.

Joseph, R. A., Mackley, A. B., Davis, C. G., Spear, M. L., & Locke, R. G. (2007). Stress in fathers of surgical neonatal intensive care unit babies. *Advances in Neonatal Care, 7*(6), 321–325.

Jubinville, J., Newburn-Cook, C., Hegadoren, K., & Lacaze-Masmonteil, T. (2012). Symptoms of acute stress disorder in mothers of premature infants. *Advances in Neonatal Care, 12*(4), 246–253.

Jung, Y. H., Lee, J., Kim, H. S., Shin, S. H., Sohn, J. A., Kim, E. K., & Choi, J. H. (2013). The efficacy of noninvasive hemoglobin measurement by pulse CO-oximetry in neonates. *Pediatric Critical Care Medicine, 14*(1), 70–73.

Kaiser, J. R., Gauss, C. H., & Williams, D. K. (2008). Tracheal suctioning is associated with prolonged disturbances of cerebral hemodynamics in very low birth weight infants. *Journal of Perinatology, 28*(1), 34–41.

Kalassian, K. G., Dremsizov, T., & Angus, D. C. (2002). Translating research evidence into clinical practice: New challenges for critical care. *Critical Care, 6*(1), 11–14.

Kamdar, B. B., Needham, D. M., & Collop, N. A. (2012). Sleep deprivation in critical illness: Its role in physical and psychological recovery. *Journal of Intensive Care Medicine, 27*(2), 97–111.

Kane-Urrabazo, C. (2006). Management's role in shaping organizational culture. *Journal of Nursing Management, 14*(3), 188–194.

Kaneyasu, M. (2012). Pain management, morphine administration, and outcomes in preterm infants: A review of the literature. *Neonatal Network, 31*(1), 21–30.

Kant, I. (1959). *Foundations of the metaphysics of morals.* New York, NY: Macmillan.

Kapellou, O. (2011, April 5). Blood sampling in infants (reducing pain and morbidity). *Clinical Evidence.* Retrieved from http://www.ncbi.nlm.nih.gov/pmc/articles/PMC3275293

Karr-Morse, R., & Wiley, M. S. (2012). *Scared sick: The role of childhood trauma in adult disease.* New York, NY: Basic Books.

Kessler, R. C., Aguilar-Gaxiola, S., Alonso, J., Chatterji, S., Lee, S., Ormel, J., . . . Wang, P. S. (2009). The global burden of mental disorders: An update from the WHO World Mental Health (WMH) surveys. *Epidemiologia e Psichiatria Sociale, 18*(1), 23–33.

Kindig, D., & Stoddart, G. (2003). What is population health? *American Journal of Public Health, 93*(3), 380–383.

Kirk, A. T., Alder, S. C., & King, J. D. (2007). Cue-based oral feeding clinical pathway results in earlier attainment of full oral feeding in premature infants. *Journal of Perinatology, 27*(9), 572–578.

Koloroutis, M. (2004). *Relationship-based care: A model for transforming practice.* Minneapolis, MN: Creative Health Care Management.

Konturek, P. C., Brzozowski, T., & Konturek, S. J. (2011). Stress and the gut: Pathophysiology, clinical consequences, diagnostic approach and treatment options. *Journal of Physiology and Pharmacology, 62*(6), 591–599.

Korsch, B. M. (1978). Issues in humanizing care for children. *American Journal of Public Health, 68*(9), 831–832.

Kristoffersen, L., Skogvoll, E., & Hafström, M. (2011). Pain reduction on insertion of a feeding tube in preterm infants: A randomized controlled trial. *Pediatrics, 127*(6), e1449–e1454.

Krueger, C., Parker, L., Chiu, S.-H., & Theriaque, D. (2010). Maternal voice and short-term outcomes in preterm infants. *Developmental Psychobiology, 52*(2), 205–212.

Kumar, P., Denson, S. E., & Mancuso, T. J.; Committee on Fetus and Newborn, Section on Anesthesiology and Pain Medicine. (2010). Premedication for non-emergency endotracheal intubation in the neonate. *Pediatrics, 125*(3), 608–615.

Kuo, D. Z., Houtrow, A. J., Arango, P., Kuhlthau, K. A., Simmons, J. M., & Neff, J. M. (2012). Family-centered care: Current applications and future directions in pediatric health care. *Maternal and Child Health Journal, 16*(2), 297–305.

Lago, P., Garetti, E., Merazzi, D., Pieragostini, L., Ancora, G., Pirelli, A., & Bellieni, C. V.; Pain Study Group of the Italian Society of Neonatology. (2009). Guidelines for procedural pain in the newborn. *Acta Paediatrica, 98*(6), 932–939.

Lai, M. C., & Huang, L. T. (2011). Effects of early life stress on neuroendocrine and neurobehavior: Mechanisms and implications. *Pediatrics and Neonatology, 52*(3), 122–129.

Lai, T. T., & Bearer, C. F. (2008). Iatrogenic environmental hazards in the neonatal intensive care unit. *Clinics in Perinatology, 35*(1), 163–181, ix.

Lajud, N., Roque, A., Cajero, M., Gutiérrez-Ospina, G., & Torner, L. (2012). Periodic maternal separation decreases hippocampal neurogenesis without affecting basal corticosterone during the stress hyporesponsive period, but alters HPA axis and coping behavior in adulthood. *Psychoneuroendocrinology, 37*(3), 410–420.

Lampl, M., & Johnson, M. L. (2011). Infant growth in length follows prolonged sleep and increased naps. *Sleep, 34*(5), 641–650.

Larsson, B. A., Norman, M., Bjerring, P., Egekvist, H., Lagercrantz, H., & Olsson, G. L. (1996). Regional variations in skin perfusion and skin thickness may contribute to varying efficacy of topical, local anaesthetics in neonates. *Paediatric Anaesthesia, 6*(2), 107–110.

Lasiuk, G. C., Comeau, T., & Newburn-Cook, C. (2013). Unexpected: An interpretive description of parental traumas associated with preterm birth. *BMC Pregnancy and Childbirth, 13*(Suppl. 1), S13.

Latimer, M. A., Johnston, C. C., Ritchie, J. A., Clarke, S. P., & Gilin, D. (2009). Factors affecting delivery of evidence-based procedural pain care in hospitalized neonates. *Journal of Obstetric, Gynecologic, and Neonatal Nursing, 38*(2), 182–194.

Lau, C., Geddes, D., Mizuno, K., & Schaal, B. (2012). The development of oral feeding skills in infants. *International Journal of Pediatrics, 2012*, 572341.

Leape, L. L., Shore, M. F., Dienstag, J. L., Mayer, R. J., Edgman-Levitan, S., Meyer, G. S., & Healy, G. B. (2012). Perspective: A culture of respect, part 1: The nature and causes of disrespectful behavior by physicians. *Academic Medicine, 87*(7), 845–852.

Lee, H. K. (2002). Effects of sponge bathing on vagal tone and behavioural responses in premature infants. *Journal of Clinical Nursing, 11*(4), 510–519.

Lefaiver, C. A., Lawlor-Klean, P., Welling, R., Smith, J., Waszak, L., & Micek, W. T. (2009). Using evidence to improve care for the vulnerable neonatal population. *The Nursing Clinics of North America, 44*(1), 131–144, xii.

Lehr, V. T., & Taddio, A. (2007). Topical anesthesia in neonates: Clinical practices and practical considerations. *Seminars in Perinatology, 31*(5), 323–329.

Lehtonen, L., & Martin, R. J. (2004). Ontogeny of sleep and awake states in relation to breathing in preterm infants. *Seminars in Neonatology, 9*(3), 229–238.

Lewandowski, A. J., Augustine, D., Lamata, P., Davis, E. F., Lazdam, M., Francis, J.,...Leeson, P. (2013). Preterm heart in adult life: Cardiovascular magnetic resonance reveals distinct differences in left ventricular mass, geometry, and function. *Circulation, 127*(2), 197–206.

Liaw, J. J., Yang, L., Chou, H. L., Yang, M. H., & Chao, S. C. (2010). Relationships between nurse care-giving behaviours and preterm infant responses during bathing: A preliminary study. *Journal of Clinical Nursing, 19*(1–2), 89–99.

Liaw, J. J., Yang, L., Hua, Y. M., Chang, P. W., Teng, C. C., & Li, C. C. (2012). Preterm infants' biobehavioral responses to caregiving and positioning over 24 hours in a neonatal unit in Taiwan. *Research in Nursing & Health, 35*(6), 634–646.

Liaw, J. J., Yang, L., Katherine Wang, K. W., Chen, C. M., Chang, Y. C., & Yin, T. (2012). Non-nutritive sucking and facilitated tucking relieve preterm infant pain during heel-stick procedures: A prospective, randomised controlled crossover trial. *International Journal of Nursing Studies, 49*(3), 300–309.

Liaw, J. J., Yang, L., Lee, C. M., Fan, H. C., Chang, Y. C., & Cheng, L. P. (2013). Effects of combined use of non-nutritive sucking, oral sucrose, and facilitated tucking on infant behavioural states across heel-stick procedures: A prospective, randomised controlled trial. *International Journal of Nursing Studies, 50*(7), 883–894.

Liaw, J. J., Yang, L., Yuh, Y. S., & Yin, T. (2006). Effects of tub bathing procedures on preterm infants' behavior. *The Journal of Nursing Research, 14*(4), 297–305.

Limperopoulos, C., Gauvreau, K. K., O'Leary, H., Moore, M., Bassan, H., Eichenwald, E. C.,...du Plessis, A. J. (2008). Cerebral hemodynamic changes during intensive care of preterm infants. *Pediatrics, 122*(5), e1006–e1013.

Lipchock, S. V., Reed, D. R., & Mennella, J. A. (2011). The gustatory and olfactory systems during infancy: Implications for development of feeding behaviors in the high-risk neonate. *Clinics in Perinatology, 38*(4), 627–641.

Loewy, J., Stewart, K., Dassler, A. M., Telsey, A., & Homel, P. (2013). The effects of music therapy on vital signs, feeding, and sleep in premature infants. *Pediatrics, 131*(5), 902–918.

Loizzo, A., Loizzo, S., & Capasso, A. (2009). Neurobiology of pain in children: An overview. *The Open Biochemistry Journal, 3*, 18–25.

Longo, J. (2010). Combating disruptive behaviors: Strategies to promote a healthy work environment. *The Online Journal of Issues in Nursing, 15*(1), Manuscript 5.

Low, L. A., & Schweinhardt, P. (2012). Early life adversity as a risk factor for fibromyalgia in later life. *Pain Research and Treatment, 2012*, 140832.

Lown, B. A., Rosen, J., & Marttila, J. (2011). An agenda for improving compassionate care: A survey shows about half of patients say such care is missing. *Health Affairs, 30*(9), 1772–1778.

Ludington-Hoe, S. M., Johnson, M. W., Morgan, K., Lewis, T., Gutman, J., Wilson, P. D., & Scher, M. S. (2006). Neurophysiologic assessment of neonatal sleep organization: Preliminary results of a randomized, controlled trial of skin contact with preterm infants. *Pediatrics, 117*(5), e909–e923.

Ludington-Hoe, S. M., Morgan, K., & Abouelfettoh, A. (2008). A clinical guideline for implementation of kangaroo care with premature infants of 30 or more weeks' postmenstrual age. *Advances in Neonatal Care, 8*(3S), S3–S23.

Ludwig, S. M., & Waitzman, K. A. (2007). Changing feeding documentation to reflect infant-driven feeding practice. *Newborn and Infant Nursing Reviews, 7*(3), 155–160.

Lund, C. H., & Osborne, J. W. (2004). Validity and reliability of the neonatal skin condition score. *Journal of Obstetric, Gynecologic, and Neonatal Nursing, 33*(3), 320–327.

Lund, L. K., Vik, T., Lohaugen, G. C. C., Skarnes, J., Brubakk, A.-M., & Indredavik, M. S. (2012). Mental health, quality of life and social relations in young adults born with low birth weight. *Health and Quality of Life Outcomes, 10*, 146. Retrieved from http://www.hqlo.com/content/10/1/146

Lundqvist, P., & Jakobsson, L. (2003). Swedish men's experiences of becoming fathers to their preterm infants. *Neonatal Network, 22*(6), 25–31.

Malusky, S., & Donze, A. (2011). Neutral head positioning in premature infants for intraventricular hemorrhage prevention: An evidence-based review. *Neonatal Network, 30*(6), 381–396.

Marco, E. M., Macrì, S., & Laviola, G. (2011). Critical age windows for neurodevelopmental psychiatric disorders: Evidence from animal models. *Neurotoxicity Research, 19*(2), 286–307.

Marino, B. S., Lipkin, P. H., Newburger, J. W., Peacock, G., Gerdes, M., Gaynor, J. W., … Mahle, W. T.; American Heart Association Congenital Heart Defects Committee, Council on Cardiovascular Disease in the Young, Council on Cardiovascular Nursing, and Stroke Council. (2012). Neurodevelopmental outcomes in children with congenital heart disease: Evaluation and management: A scientific statement from the American Heart Association. *Circulation, 126*(9), 1143–1172.

Maroney, D. I. (2003). Recognizing the potential effect of stress and trauma on premature infants in the NICU: How are outcomes affected? *Journal of Perinatology, 23*(8), 679–683.

Mata, L. (1978). Breast-feeding: Main promoter of infant health. *The American Journal of Clinical Nutrition, 31*(11), 2058–2065.

Mathers, C. D., & Loncar, D. (2006). Projections of global mortality and burden of disease from 2002 to 2030. *PLoS Medicine, 3*(11), e442.

Maton, P., & Francoise, A. (2011, June 18). *Global care program*. Oral presentation at the XXVII Rencontre de Néonatologie (Rocourt): The Neonatal Environment, Rocourt, Belgium.

Maton, P., Marguglio, A., Marion, W., Langhendries, J.-P., Jonlet, M.-H., Gibbins, S., … Francoise, A. (2010, February). *Developmental care practice improvement in a single institution using a standardized team approach: Clinical outcomes at discharge*. Poster presented at the 23rd Annual Gravens Conference on the Physical and Developmental Environment of the High Risk Infant, Clearwater Beach, FL.

McCabe, K., Blucker, R., Gillaspy, J. A., Cherry, A., Mignogna, M., Roddenberry, A.,...Gillaspy, S. R. (2012). Reliability of the postpartum depression screening scale in the neonatal intensive care unit. *Nursing Research, 61*(6), 441–445.

McCullough, S., Halton, T., Mowbray, D., & Macfarlane, P. I. (2008). Lingual sucrose reduces the pain response to nasogastric tube insertion: A randomised clinical trial. *Archives of Disease in Childhood, 93*(2), F100–F103.

McDonald, J., Jayasuriya, R., & Harris, M. F. (2012). The influence of power dynamics and trust on multidisciplinary collaboration: A qualitative case study of type 2 diabetes mellitus. *BMC Health Services Research, 12*, 63.

McEwen, B. S. (2011, September). Effects of stress on the developing brain. *Cerebrum*. Retrieved from http://dana.org/news/cerebrum/detail.aspx?id=34202

McEwen, B. S., & Gianaros, P. J. (2011). Stress- and allostasis-induced brain plasticity. *Annual Review of Medicine, 62*, 431–445.

McGuckin, M., Waterman, R., & Govednik, J. (2009). Hand hygiene compliance rates in the United States—A one-year multicenter collaboration using product/volume usage measurement and feedback. *American Journal of Medical Quality, 24*(3), 205–213.

McLeroy, K. R., & Crump, C. E. (1994, March 22). Health promotion and disease prevention: A historical perspective. *Generations, 18*(1), 9–17.

McManus, B. M., & Capistran, P. S. (2008). A case presentation of early intervention with dolichocephaly in the NICU: Collaboration between the primary nursing team and the developmental care specialist. *Neonatal Network, 27*(5), 307–315.

McMullen, S. L. (2013). Transitioning premature infants supine: State of the science. *The American Journal of Maternal Child Nursing, 38*(1), 8–12; quiz 13.

McMullen, S. L., Lipke, B., & LeMura, C. (2009). Sudden infant death syndrome prevention: A model program for NICUs. *Neonatal Network, 28*(1), 7–12.

McPherson, C. (2012). Sedation and analgesia in mechanically ventilated preterm neonates: Continue standard of care or experiment? *The Journal of Pediatric Pharmacology and Therapeutics, 17*(4), 351–364.

Meadow, W., & Lantos, J. (2009). Moral reflections on neonatal intensive care. *Pediatrics, 123*(2), 595–597.

Meier, P. P., Engstrom, J. L., Patel, A. L., Jegier, B. J., & Bruns, N. E. (2010). Improving the use of human milk during and after the NICU stay. *Clinics in Perinatology, 37*(1), 217–245.

Melnyk, B. M., Feinstein, N. F., Alpert-Gillis, L., Fairbanks, E., Crean, H. F., Sinkin, R. A.,...Gross, S. J. (2006). Reducing premature infants' length of stay and improving parents' mental health outcomes with the Creating Opportunities for Parent Empowerment (COPE) neonatal intensive care unit program: A randomized, controlled trial. *Pediatrics, 118*(5), e1414–e1427.

Menon, G., & McIntosh, N. (2008). How should we manage pain in ventilated neonates? *Neonatology, 93*(4), 316–323.

Mewes, A. U., Zöllei, L., Hüppi, P. S., Als, H., McAnulty, G. B., Inder, T. E.,... Warfield, S. K. (2007). Displacement of brain regions in preterm infants with non-synostotic dolichocephaly investigated by MRI. *NeuroImage, 36*(4), 1074–1085.

Milgrom, J., Newnham, C., Martin, P. R., Anderson, P. J., Doyle, L. W., Hunt, R. W.,... Gemmill, A. W. (2013). Early communication in preterm infants following intervention in the NICU. *Early Human Development, 89*(9), 755–762.

Mitchell, A. J., Green, A., Jeffs, D. A., & Roberson, P. K. (2011). Physiologic effects of retinopathy of prematurity screening examinations. *Advances in Neonatal Care, 11*(4), 291–297.

Monterosso, L., Kristjanson, L. J., Cole, J., & Evans, S. F. (2003). Effect of postural supports on neuromotor function in very preterm infants to term equivalent age. *Journal of Paediatrics and Child Health, 39*(3), 197–205.

Montirosso, R., Del Prete, A., Bellù, R., Tronick, E., & Borgatti, R.; Neonatal Adequate Care for Quality of Life (NEO-ACQUA) Study Group. (2012). Level of NICU quality of developmental care and neurobehavioral performance in very preterm infants. *Pediatrics, 129*(5), e1129–e1137.

Moore, T. A., Berger, A. M., & Wilson, M. E. (2012). A new way of thinking about complications of prematurity. *Biological Research for Nursing*. Advance online publication. doi:10.1177/1099800412461563

Mörelius, E., Hellström-Westas, L., Carlén, C., Norman, E., & Nelson, N. (2006). Is a nappy change stressful to neonates? *Early Human Development, 82*(10), 669–676.

Morningstar, M. W., Pettibon, B. R., Schlappi, H., Schlappi, M., & Ireland, T. V. (2005). Reflex control of the spine and posture: A review of the literature from a chiropractic perspective. *Chiropractic & Osteopathy, 13*, 16.

Mosqueda, R., Castilla, Y., Perapoch, J., Lora, D., López-Maestro, M., & Pallás, C. (2013). Necessary resources and barriers perceived by professionals in the implementation of the NIDCAP. *Early Human Development, 89*(9), 649–653.

Naef, R. (2006). Bearing witness: A moral way of engaging in the nurse-person relationship. *Nursing Philosophy, 7*(3), 146–156.

Nakos, G. (2012). Sleep deprivation in ICU. *Minerva Anestesiologica, 78*(4), 395–396.

Nanavati, R. N., Balan, R., & Kabra, N. S. (2013). Effect of kangaroo mother care expressed breast milk administration on pain associated with removal of adhesive tapes in very low birth weight neonates: A randomized controlled trial. *Indian Pediatrics*. May 5. pii: S097475591200346. [Epub ahead of print]

National Child Traumatic Stress Network Complex Trauma Task Force. (2003). *Complex trauma in children and adolescents* (White Paper). Retrieved from http://www.nctsn.org/sites/default/files/assets/pdfs/ComplexTrauma_All.pdf

National Research Council. (2007). *Preterm birth: Causes, consequences, and prevention*. Washington, DC: The National Academies Press.

National Scientific Council on the Developing Child. (2005). *Excessive stress disrupts the architecture of the developing brain* (Working Paper No. 3). Retrieved from http://www.developingchild.net

Naughton, K. A. (2013). The combined use of sucrose and nonnutritive sucking for procedural pain in both term and preterm neonates: An integrative review of the literature. *Advances in Neonatal Care, 13*(1), 9–19; quiz 20.

Ness, M. J., Davis, D. M., & Carey, W. A. (2013). Neonatal skin care: A concise review. *International Journal of Dermatology, 52*(1), 14–22.

Newland, L., L'huillier, M. W., & Petrey, B. (2013). Implementation of cue-based feeding in a level III NICU. *Neonatal Network, 32*(2), 132–137.

Newnham, C. A., Inder, T. E., & Milgrom, J. (2009). Measuring preterm cumulative stressors within the NICU: The Neonatal Infant Stressor Scale. *Early Human Development, 85*(9), 549–555.

Nightingale, F. (1915). *Florence Nightingale to her nurses.* London, UK: Macmillan.

Nijhuis, J. G., Prechtl, H. F., Martin, C. B., & Bots, R. S. (1982). Are there behavioural states in the human fetus? *Early Human Development, 6*(2), 177–195.

Nimbalkar, S., Sinojia, A., & Dongara, A. (2013). Reduction of neonatal pain following administration of 25% lingual dextrose: A randomized control trial. *Journal of Tropical Pediatrics, 59*(3), 223–225.

Niwa, M., Matsumoto, Y., Mouri, A., Ozaki, N., & Nabeshima, T. (2011). Vulnerability in early life to changes in the rearing environment plays a crucial role in the aetiopathology of psychiatric disorders. *The International Journal of Neuropsychopharmacology, 14*(4), 459–477.

Nolan, P. J. (2013). The meaning of persons in medicine. *Journal of Healthcare Leadership, 5*, 31–33.

Noonan, C., Quigley, S., & Curley, M. A. (2011). Using the Braden Q Scale to Predict Pressure Ulcer Risk in pediatric patients. *Journal of Pediatric Nursing, 26*(6), 566–575.

Nosarti, C., Reichenberg, A., Murray, R. M., Cnattingius, S., Lambe, M. P., Yin, L.,...& Hultman, C. M. (2012). Preterm birth and psychiatric disorders in young adult life. *Archives of General Psychiatry, 69*(6), E1–E8.

Nummenmaa, L., Glerean, E., Viinikainen, M., Jääskeläinen, I. P., Hari, R., & Sams, M. (2012). Emotions promote social interaction by synchronizing brain activity across individuals. *Proceedings of the National Academy of Sciences of the United States of America, 109*(24), 9599–9604.

Nye, C. (2008). Transitioning premature infants from gavage to breast. *Neonatal Network, 27*(1), 7–13.

Nyqvist, K. H., Anderson, G. C., Bergman, N., Cattaneo, A., Charpak, N., Davanzo, R.,...Widström, A. M. (2010). Towards universal Kangaroo Mother Care: Recommendations and report from the First European conference and Seventh International Workshop on Kangaroo Mother Care. *Acta Paediatrica, 99*(6), 820–826.

Ogawa, S., Ogihara, T., Fujiwara, E., Ito, K., Nakano, M., Nakayama, S.,...Tamai, H. (2005). Venepuncture is preferable to heel lance for blood sampling in term neonates. *Archives of Disease in Childhood, 90*(5), F432–F436.

Ohlinger, J., Brown, M. S., Laudert, S., Swanson, S., & Fofah, O.; CARE Group. (2003). Development of potentially better practices for the neonatal intensive care unit as a culture of collaboration: Communication, accountability, respect, and empowerment. *Pediatrics, 111*(4, Pt. 2), e471–e481.

Osorio, M. J., Hertle, R. W., Painter, M., & Hinch, K. (2009). Pupillary light reflexes in premature infants prior to 30 weeks postmenstrual age. *Journal of American Association for Pediatric Ophthalmology and Strabismus, 13*(6), 608–609.

Pandey, M., Datta, V., & Rehan, H. S. (2013). Role of sucrose in reducing painful response to orogastric tube insertion in preterm neonates. *Indian Journal of Pediatrics, 80*(6), 476–482.

Paquin, S. O. (2011). Social justice advocacy in nursing: What is it? How do we get there? *Creative Nursing, 17*(2), 63–67.

Parrotta, C., Riley, W., & Meredith, L. (2012). Utilizing leadership to achieve high reliability in the delivery of perinatal care. *Journal of Healthcare Leadership, 4,* 157–163.

Pechtel, P., & Pizzagalli, D. A. (2011). Effects of early life stress on cognitive and affective function: An integrated review of human literature. *Psychopharmacology, 214*(1), 55–70.

Peirano, P., Algarín, C., & Uauy, R. (2003). Sleep-wake states and their regulatory mechanisms throughout early human development. *The Journal of Pediatrics, 143*(4, Suppl.), S70–S79.

Peirano, P. D., & Algarín, C. R. (2007). Sleep in brain development. *Biological Research, 40*(4), 471–478.

Peixoto, P. V., de Araújo, M. A., Kakehashi, T. Y., & Pinheiro, E. M. (2011). [Sound pressure levels in the neonatal intensive care unit]. *Revista da Escola de Enfermagem da U S P, 45*(6), 1309–1314.

Pellicer, A., Gayá, F., Madero, R., Quero, J., & Cabañas, F. (2002). Noninvasive continuous monitoring of the effects of head position on brain hemodynamics in ventilated infants. *Pediatrics, 109*(3), 434–440.

Pepper, D., Rempel, G., Austin, W., Ceci, C., & Hendson, L. (2012). More than information: A qualitative study of parents' perspectives on neonatal intensive care at the extremes of prematurity. *Advances in Neonatal Care, 12*(5), 303–309.

Perrone, S., Tataranno, M. L., Negro, S., Cornacchione, S., Longini, M., Proietti, F., ... Buonocore, G. (2012). May oxidative stress biomarkers in cord blood predict the occurrence of necrotizing enterocolitis in preterm infants? *Journal of Maternal-Fetal & Neonatal Medicine, 25*(Suppl. 1), 128–131.

Perry, B. D., Pollard, R. A., Blakely, T. L., Baker, W. L., & Vigilante, D. (1995). Childhood trauma, the neurobiology of adaptation, and "use-dependent" development of the brain: How "states" become "traits." *Infant Mental Health Journal, 16*(4), 271–291.

Peters, J. W., Schouw, R., Anand, K. J., van Dijk, M., Duivenvoorden, H. J., & Tibboel, D. (2005). Does neonatal surgery lead to increased pain sensitivity in later childhood? *Pain, 114*(3), 444–454.

Pichler, G., van Boetzelar, M. C., Müller, W., & Urlesberger, B. (2001). Effect of tilting on cerebral hemodynamics in preterm and term infants. *Biology of the Neonate, 80*(3), 179–185.

Pickler, R. H. (2004). A model of feeding readiness for preterm infants. *Neonatal Intensive Care, 17*(4), 31–36.

Pillai Riddell, R., Racine, N., Turcotte, K., Uman, L., Horton, R., Din Osmun, L.,...Lisi, D. (2011). Nonpharmacological management of procedural pain in infants and young children: An abridged Cochrane review. *Pain Research & Management, 16*(5), 321–330.

Pimenta, H. P., Moreira, M. E., Rocha, A. D., Gomes Jr., S. C., Pinto, L. W., & Lucena, S. L. (2008). Effects of non-nutritive sucking and oral stimulation on breast-feeding rates for preterm, low birth weight infants: A randomized clinical trial. *Jornal de Pediatria, 84*(5), 423–427.

Pinheiro, E. M., Guinsburg, R., Nabuco, M. A., & Kakehashi, T. Y. (2011). Noise at the neonatal intensive care unit and inside the incubator. *Revista Latino-Americana de Enfermagem, 19*(5), 1214–1221.

Puchalski, M., & Hummel, P. (2002). The reality of neonatal pain. *Advances in Neonatal Care, 2*(5), 233–244; quiz 245.

Pyner, S. (2009). Neurochemistry of the paraventricular nucleus of the hypo-thalamus: Implications for cardiovascular regulation. *Journal of Chemical Neuroanatomy, 38*(3), 197–208.

Quinn, D., Newton, N., & Piecuch, R. (2005). Effect of less frequent bathing on premature infant skin. *Journal of Obstetric, Gynecologic, and Neonatal Nursing, 34*(6), 741–746.

Quinn, M. (2008). Oral aversion. In D. Brodsky & M. A. Ouellette (Eds.), *Primary care of the premature infant* (1st ed., pp. 101–104). Philadelphia, PA: Saunders Elsevier.

Raju, T. N., Suresh, G., & Higgins, R. D. (2011). Patient safety in the context of neonatal intensive care: Research and educational opportunities. *Pediatric Research, 70*(1), 109–115.

Reinhard, S., & Hassmiller, S. (2012). The future of nursing: Transforming health care. *The Journal.* Retrieved from http://journal.aarpinternational.org/a/b/2012/02/The-Future-of-Nursing-Transforming-Health-Care

Reynolds, L. C., Duncan, M. M., Smith, G. C., Mathur, A., Neil, J., Inder, T., & Pineda, R. G. (2013). Parental presence and holding in the neonatal intensive care unit and associations with early neurobehavior. *Journal of Perinatology, 33*(8), 636–641.

Rifkin-Graboi, A., Borelli, J. L., & Enlow, M. B. (2009). Neurobiology of stress in infancy. In C. H. Zeanah, Jr. (Ed.), *Handbook of infant mental health* (3rd ed., pp. 40–58). New York, NY: Guilford Press.

Rivkees, S. A., Mayes, L., Jacobs, H., & Gross, I. (2004). Rest-activity patterns of pre-mature infants are regulated by cycled lighting. *Pediatrics, 113*(4), 833–839.

Robinson, J., & Fielder, A. R. (1990). Pupillary diameter and reaction to light in preterm neonates. *Archives of Disease in Childhood, 65*(1 Spec. No.), 35–38.

Roisman, G. I., & Fraley, R. C. (2012). The legacy of early interpersonal experi-ence. *Advances in Child Development and Behavior, 42,* 79–112.

Ross, E. S., & Philbin, M. K. (2011). Supporting oral feeding in fragile infants: An evidence-based method for quality bottle-feedings of preterm, ill, and fragile infants. *The Journal of Perinatal & Neonatal Nursing, 25*(4), 349–357; quiz 358.

Rossman, B., Kratovil, A. L., Greene, M. M., Engstrom, J. L., & Meier, P. P. (2013). "I have faith in my milk": The meaning of milk for mothers of very low birth weight infants hospitalized in the neonatal intensive care unit. *Journal of Human Lactation, 29*(3), 359–365.

Saigal, S., & Doyle, L. W. (2008). An overview of mortality and sequelae of preterm birth from infancy to adulthood. *Lancet, 371*(9608), 261–269.

Samra, H. A., & McGrath, J. M. (2009). Pain management during retinopathy of prematurity eye examinations: A systematic review. *Advances in Neonatal Care, 9*(3), 99–110.

Sandberg, K. L., Brynjarsson, H., & Hjalmarson, O. (2011). Transcutaneous blood gas monitoring during neonatal intensive care. *Acta Paediatrica, 100*(5), 676–679.

Schechter, D. S., & Willheim, E. (2009). Disturbances of attachment and parental psychopathology in early childhood. *Child and Adolescent Psychiatric Clinics of North America, 18*(3), 665–686.

Scher, M. S., Johnson, M. W., & Holditch-Davis, D. (2005). Cyclicity of neonatal sleep behaviors at 25 to 30 weeks' postconceptional age. *Pediatric Research, 57*(6), 879–882.

Scher, M. S., Ludington-Hoe, S., Kaffashi, F., Johnson, M. W., Holditch-Davis, D., & Loparo, K. A. (2009). Neurophysiologic assessment of brain maturation after an 8-week trial of skin-to-skin contact on preterm infants. *Clinical Neurophysiology, 120*(10), 1812–1818.

Schoenhofer, S. O. (2002). Choosing personhood: Intentionality and the theory of nursing as caring. *Holistic Nursing Practice, 16*(4), 36–40.

Schore, A. N. (2001a). Effects of a secure attachment relationship on right brain development, affect regulation, and infant mental health. *Infant Mental Health Journal, 22*(1–2), 7–66.

Schore, A. N. (2001b). The effects of early relational trauma on right brain development, affect regulation, and infant mental health. *Infant Mental Health Journal, 22*(1–2), 201–269.

Schweitzer, M., Gilpin, L., & Frampton, S. (2004). Healing spaces: Elements of environmental design that make an impact on health. *Journal of Alternative and Complementary Medicine, 10*(Suppl. 1), S71–S83.

Seifert, P. C., & Hickman, D. S. (2005). Enhancing patient safety in a healing environment. *Topics in Advanced Practice Nursing eJournal, 5*(1). Retrieved from http://www.medscape.com/viewarticle/499690_6

Selanders, L. C. (2005). Leading through theory: Nightingale's environmental adaptation theory of nursing practice. In B. M. Dossey, L. C. Selanders, D.-M. Beck, & A. Attewell (Eds.), *Florence Nightingale today: Healing, leadership, global action* (pp. 97–114). Silver Springs, MD: nursebooks.org.

Selanders, L. C. (2010). The power of environmental adaptation: Florence Nightingale's original theory for nursing practice. *Journal of Holistic Nursing, 28*(1), 81–88.

Seltzer, L. J., Ziegler, T. E., & Pollak, S. D. (2010). Social vocalizations can release oxytocin in humans. *Proceedings. Biological Sciences/The Royal Society, 277*(1694), 2661–2666.

Shah, V. S., Taddio, A., Bennett, S., & Speidel, B. D. (1997). Neonatal pain response to heel stick vs venepuncture for routine blood sampling. *Archives of Disease in Childhood, 77*(2), F143–F144.

Shaw, R. J., Bernard, R. S., Deblois, T., Ikuta, L. M., Ginzburg, K., & Koopman, C. (2009). The relationship between acute stress disorder and posttraumatic stress disorder in the neonatal intensive care unit. *Psychosomatics, 50*(2), 131–137.

Siegel, D. J. (2010). *The mindful therapist: A clinician's guide to mindsight and neural integration.* New York, NY: W. W. Norton & Company.

Simons, S. H., van Dijk, M., Anand, K. S., Roofthooft, D., van Lingen, R. A., & Tibboel, D. (2003). Do we still hurt newborn babies? A prospective study of procedural pain and analgesia in neonates. *Archives of Pediatrics & Adolescent Medicine, 157*(11), 1058–1064.

Skene, C., Franck, L., Curtis, P., & Gerrish, K. (2012). Parental involvement in neonatal comfort care. *Journal of Obstetric, Gynecologic, and Neonatal Nursing, 41*(6), 786–797.

Slater, L., Asmerom, Y., Boskovic, D. S., Bahjri, K., Plank, M. S., Angeles, K. R.,...Angeles, D. M. (2012). Procedural pain and oxidative stress in premature neonates. *The Journal of Pain, 13*(6), 590–597.

Smith, G. C., Gutovich, J., Smyser, C., Pineda, R., Newnham, C., Tjoeng, T. H.,...Inder, T. (2011). Neonatal intensive care unit stress is associated with brain development in preterm infants. *Annals of Neurology, 70*(4), 541–549.

Smith, S. L., Lux, R., Haley, S., Slater, H., Beachy, J., Beechy, J., & Moyer-Mileur, L. J. (2013). The effect of massage on heart rate variability in preterm infants. *Journal of Perinatology, 33*(1), 59–64.

Solodkin, A., & Stern, H. (2012). Fragmentation and unpredictability of early-life experience in mental disorders. *American Journal of Psychiatry, 169,* 907–915.

Sourkes, B. M. (2007). Armfuls of time: The psychological experience of the child with a life-threatening illness. *Medical Principles and Practice, 16*(Suppl. 1), 37–41.

Spence Laschinger, H. K., Leiter, M., Day, A., & Gilin, D. (2009). Workplace empowerment, incivility, and burnout: Impact on staff nurse recruitment and retention outcomes. *Journal of Nursing Management, 17*(3), 302–311.

Spenrath, M. A., Clarke, M. E., & Kutcher, S. (2011). The science of brain and biological development: Implications for mental health research, practice and policy. *Journal of Canadian Academy of Child and Adolescent Psychiatry, 20*(4), 298–304.

Spitz, R. A. (1945). Hospitalism: An inquiry into the genesis of psychiatric conditions in early childhood. *The Psychoanalytic Study of the Child, 1,* 53–74.

Spitz, R. A. (1951). The psychogenic diseases in infancy—An attempt at their etiologic classification. *Psychoanalytic Study of the Child, 6,* 255–275.

Srinivasan, V. (2012). Stress hyperglycemia in pediatric critical illness: The intensive care unit adds to the stress! *Journal of Diabetes Science and Technology, 6*(1), 37–47.

Standley, J. (2012). Music therapy research in the NICU: An updated meta-analysis. *Neonatal Network, 31*(5), 311–316.

Sullivan, M. C., Hawes, K., Winchester, S. B., & Miller, R. J. (2008). Developmental origins theory from prematurity to adult disease. *Journal of Obstetric, Gynecologic, and Neonatal Nursing, 37*(2), 158–164.

Sweeney, J. K., & Gutierrez, T. (2002). Musculoskeletal implications of preterm infant positioning in the NICU. *The Journal of Perinatal & Neonatal Nursing, 16*(1), 58–70.

Sweeney, J. K., & Gutierrez, T. (2010). The dynamic continuum of motor and musculoskeletal development. In C. Kenner & J. M. McGrath (Eds.), *Developmental care of newborns and infants: A guide for health professionals* (2nd ed., pp. 235–244). Glenview, IL: National Association of Neonatal Nurses.

Tarullo, A. R., Balsam, P. D., & Fifer, W. P. (2011). Sleep and infant learning. *Infant and Child Development, 20*(1), 35–46.

Taylor, D. L., Edwards, A. D., & Mehmet, H. (1999). Oxidative metabolism, apoptosis and perinatal brain injury. *Brain Pathology, 9*(1), 93–117.

Telofski, L. S., Morello, A. P., Mack Correa, M. C., & Stamatas, G. N. (2012). The infant skin barrier: Can we preserve, protect, and enhance the barrier? *Dermatology Research and Practice, 2012*, 198789.

Thibeau, S., & Boudreaux, C. (2013). Exploring the use of mothers' own milk as oral care for mechanically ventilated very low-birth-weight preterm infants. *Advances in Neonatal Care, 13*(3), 190–197.

Thomson, G., Moran, V. H., Axelin, A., Dykes, F., & Flacking, R. (2013). Integrating a sense of coherence into the neonatal environment. *BMC Pediatrics, 13*, 84.

Titler, M. G. (2008). The evidence for evidence-based practice implementation. In R. G. Hughes (Ed.), *Patient safety and quality: An evidence-based handbook for nurses* (pp. 113–161). Rockville, MD: Agency for Healthcare Research and Quality.

Tronick, E., & Beeghly, M. (2011). Infants' meaning-making and the development of mental health problems. *The American Psychologist, 66*(2), 107–119.

Tronick, E. Z. (1989). Emotions and emotional communication in infants. *The American Psychologist, 44*(2), 112–119.

Ubbink, D. T., Guyatt, G. H., & Vermeulen, H. (2013). Framework of policy recommendations for implementation of evidence-based practice: A systematic scoping review. *BMJ Open, 3*(1), e001881.

Ulrich, R. S. (1997). A theory of supportive design for healthcare facilities. *Journal of Healthcare Design, 9*, 3–7; discussion 21–24.

Ulrich, R. S. (2001). Effects of healthcare environmental design on medical outcomes. In A. Dilani (Ed.), *Design and health: Proceedings of the Second International Conference on Health and Design* (pp. 49–59). Stockholm, Sweden: Svensk Byggtjanst.

Uvnäs-Moberg, K. (1996). Neuroendocrinology of the mother-child interaction. *Trends in Endocrinology and Metabolism, 7*(4), 126–131.

Vaivre-Douret, L., Ennouri, K., Jrad, I., Garrec, C., & Papiernik, E. (2004). Effect of positioning on the incidence of abnormalities of muscle tone in low-risk, preterm infants. *European Journal of Paediatric Neurology, 8*(1), 21–34.

Vanderbilt, D., & Gleason, M. M. (2010). Mental health concerns of the premature infant through the lifespan. *Child and Adolescent Psychiatric Clinics of North America, 19*(2), 211–228, vii–viii.

Veenema, A. H. (2012). Toward understanding how early-life social experiences alter oxytocin- and vasopressin-regulated social behaviors. *Hormones and Behavior, 61*(3), 304–312.

Veltman, L., & Larison, K. (2007). PURE conversations: Enhancing communication and teamwork. *Journal of Healthcare Risk Management, 27*(2), 41–44.

Ventura, A. K., & Worobey, J. (2013). Early influences on the development of food preferences. *Current Biology, 23*(9), R401–R408.

Voos, K. C., Ross, G., Ward, M. J., Yohay, A. L., Osorio, S. N., & Perlman, J. M. (2011). Effects of implementing family-centered rounds (FCR) in a neonatal intensive care unit (NICU). *Journal of Maternal Fetal & Neonatal Medicine, 24*(11), 1403–1406.

Wachman, E. M., & Lahav, A. (2011). The effects of noise on preterm infants in the NICU. *Archives of Disease in Childhood, 96*(4), F305–F309.

Walden, M., & Gibbins, S. (2012). *Newborn pain assessment and management: Guideline for practice.* Glenview, IL: National Association of Neonatal Nurses.

Watson, J. (2003). Love and caring. Ethics of face and hand—an invitation to return to the heart and soul of nursing and our deep humanity. *Nursing Administration Quarterly, 27*(3), 197–202.

Watson, J. (2005). *Caring science as sacred caring.* Philadelphia, PA: F. A. Davis.

Watson, J. (2012). *Human caring science: A theory of nursing* (2nd ed.). Toronto, Ontario, Canada: Jones & Bartlett Learning.

Weisman, O., Magori-Cohen, R., Louzoun, Y., Eidelman, A. I., & Feldman, R. (2011). Sleep-wake transitions in premature neonates predict early development. *Pediatrics, 128*(4), 706–714.

Weiss, S., Goldlust, E., & Vaucher, Y. E. (2010). Improving parent satisfaction: An intervention to increase neonatal parent-provider communication. *Journal of Perinatology, 30*(6), 425–430.

Weiss, S. J., & Wilson, P. (2006). Origins of tactile vulnerability in high-risk infants. *Advances in Neonatal Care, 6*(1), 25–36.

White, R. D., Smith, J. A., & Shepley, M. M.; Committee to Establish Recommended Standards for Newborn ICU Design. (2013). Recommended standards for newborn ICU design, eighth edition. *Journal of Perinatology, 33*(Suppl. 1), S2–16.

Whit Hall, R. (2012). Anesthesia and analgesia in the NICU. *Clinics in Perinatology, 39*(1), 239–254.

Whittaker, A., Currie, A. E., Turner, M. A., Field, D. J., Mulla, H., & Pandya, H. C. (2009). Toxic additives in medication for preterm infants. *Archives of Disease in Childhood, 94*(4), F236–F240.

Wigert, H., Dellenmark, B. M., & Bry, K. (2013). Strengths and weaknesses of parent-staff communication in the NICU: A survey assessment. *BMC Pediatrics, 13*(71). Retrieved from http://www.ncbi.nlm.nih.gov/pmc/articles/PMC3651269

World Health Organization. (2008). *The global burden of disease: 2004 update.* Geneva, Switzerland: WHO Press.

World Health Organization. (2013). *Global health estimates.* Retrieved July 24, 2013, from http://www.who.int/healthinfo/global_burden_disease/en

Wu, G., Feder, A., Cohen, H., Kim, J. J., Calderon, S., Charney, D. S., & Mathé, A. A. (2013). Understanding resilience. *Frontiers in Behavioral Neuroscience, 7,* 10.

Yeğen, B. Ç. (2010). Oxytocin and hypothalamic-pituitary-adrenal axis. *Marmara Pharmaceutical Journal, 14,* 61–66.

Zimmerman, E., Keunen, K., Norton, M., & Lahav, A. (2013). Weight gain velocity in very low-birth-weight infants: Effects of exposure to biological maternal sounds. *American Journal of Perinatology, 30*(10), 863–870.

Zimmerman, E., McMahon, E., Doheny, L., Levine, P., & Lahav, A. (2012). Transmission of biological maternal sounds does not interfere with routine NICU care: Assessment of dose variability in very low birth weight infants. *Journal of Pediatric and Neonatal Individualized Medicine, 1*(1), 73–80.

Zupancic, J. A. F. (2007). A systematic review of costs associated with preterm birth. In Institute of Medicine, *Preterm birth: Causes, consequences, and prevention.* Washington, DC: The National Academies Press. Retrieved from http://www.ncbi.nlm.nih.gov/books/NBK11391

Index

Made in the USA
Lexington, KY
14 October 2016